Engineered Nanoparticles as Drug Delivery Systems

This book highlights application of nanomaterials for drug delivery, therapy, and engineering. It covers stimuli-sensitive drug delivery systems including an overview of the physical, chemical, biological, and multi-stimuli-responsive nanosystems. It also presents analysis of clinical status for different types of nanoplatforms and assesses novel applications of nanomaterials in the areas of smart delivery and drug targeting. It further discusses the advantages and disadvantages of each application of pertinent nanomaterials.

Features:

- Provides academic introduction to the uses of nanotechnology in drug delivery.
- Discusses use of nanomaterials in targeting a drug to specific tissues and cells.
- Presents an analysis of clinical status for different types of nanoplatforms.
- Covers applications in drug delivery, therapy, and engineering.
- Focuses on how novel nanotechnology-orientated methods can help improve treatment.

This book is aimed at researchers and graduate students in biomedical and biochemical engineering, pharmaceutical, chemical and bioprocess engineering, materials science, and drug delivery mechanisms.

Emerging Materials and Technologies

Series Editor
Boris I. Kharissov

The *Emerging Materials and Technologies* series is devoted to highlighting publications centered on emerging advanced materials and novel technologies. Attention is paid to those newly discovered or applied materials with potential to solve pressing societal problems and improve quality of life, corresponding to environmental protection, medicine, communications, energy, transportation, advanced manufacturing, and related areas.

The series takes into account that, under present strong demands for energy, material, and cost savings, as well as heavy contamination problems and worldwide pandemic conditions, the area of emerging materials and related scalable technologies is a highly interdisciplinary field, with the need for researchers, professionals, and academics across the spectrum of engineering and technological disciplines. The main objective of this book series is to attract more attention to these materials and technologies and invite conversation among the international R&D community.

Scanning Probe Lithography
Fundamentals, Materials, and Applications
Yu Kyoung Ryu and Javier Martinez Rodrigo

Engineered Nanoparticles as Drug Delivery Systems
Nahid Rehman and Anjana Pandey

MXene Filled Polymer Nanocomposites
Edited by Soney C George, Sharika T. Nair, and Joice Sophia Ponraj

Polymeric Biomaterials
Fabrication, Properties and Applications
Edited by Pooja Agarwal, Divya Bajpai Tripathy, Anjali Gupta, and Bijoy Kumar Kuanr

Innovations in Green Nanoscience and Nanotechnology
Synthesis, Characterization, and Applications
Edited by Shrikaant Kulkarni

Sustainable Nanomaterials for the Construction Industry
Ghasan Fahim Huseien and Kwok Wei Shah

For more information about this series, please visit: www.routledge.com/Emerging-Materials-and-Technologies/book-series/CRCEMT

Engineered Nanoparticles as Drug Delivery Systems

Nahid Rehman and Anjana Pandey

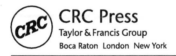

CRC Press
Taylor & Francis Group
Boca Raton London New York

CRC Press is an imprint of the
Taylor & Francis Group, an **informa** business

First edition published 2023
by CRC Press
6000 Broken Sound Parkway NW, Suite 300, Boca Raton, FL 33487-2742

and by CRC Press
4 Park Square, Milton Park, Abingdon, Oxon, OX14 4RN

CRC Press is an imprint of Taylor & Francis Group, LLC

ISBN: 9781032171760 (hbk)
ISBN: 9781032171777 (pbk)
ISBN: 9781003252122 (ebk)

DOI: 10.1201/9781003252122

Typeset in Times
by codeMantra

Contents

Authors

Nahid Rehman is currently a PhD scholar at MNNITA under the guidance of Prof. Anjana Pandey. She had completed her schooling at International Indian School in Jeddah, Saudi Arabia. Later on, she received graduation (CSJMU) in Zoology and postgraduation in Microbiology from SHUATS, India. She had worked as a Junior Research Fellow on a project at the National Institute of Immunology, New Delhi.

Anjana Pandey, currently a Professor at Motilal Nehru National Institute of Technology Allahabad (MNNITA) born in the city of New Delhi, completed her graduation, postgraduation as well as her PhD (1998) in Biochemistry from renowned Banaras Hindu University (BHU), India, and her postdoctorate from Bose Institute, Kolkata, in thrust area Molecular Microbiology (2001). Two decades have passed since her journey from lecturer to professor, starting at the University of Allahabad for 12 years and remaining at the National Institute of Technology, Allahabad, until now. Her research expertise is not just limited to her core area but extends to Environment and Health Biotechnology, Nanotechnology, and Biofuel claiming 14 honors and more than 100 publications in well-known publications.

Preface

This book highlights nanomaterials for drug delivery and therapy that present recent advances in nanobiomaterials and their critical applications in drug delivery, therapy, and engineering. Drug delivery using nanomaterials covers recent advances in the Area of stimuli-sensitive drug delivery systems, providing an up-to-date overview of the physical, chemical, biological, and multi-stimuli-responsive nanosystems. Additionally, the book also presents an analysis of clinical status for different types of nanoplatforms; also, it shows how the use of nanomaterials can help target a drug to specific tissues and cells. The book's content reconnoiters the development of stimuli-responsive drug delivery systems to platform how stimuli-responsive nanosystems are used in a variety of therapies, including camptothecin delivery, diabetes, and cancer therapy. It focuses on the implications of these nanocarriers in drug delivery and includes a detailed classification of nano-ionized drug particles, polymeric nanoparticles, and hydrophobic nanoparticles. This book assesses novel applications of nanomaterials in smart delivery and drug targeting using nanotechnology and discusses the advantages and disadvantages of each application. It also provides an academic introduction to the uses of nanotechnology in drug delivery and targeting and explores novel opportunities and ideas for developing and improving nanoscale drug delivery systems.

The book offers pharmaceutical insights, ascertaining the development of nanobiomaterials and their interaction with the human body. The book's content explains how nanomaterials are used in various treatments and therapies. This book offers a broad, overseas perspective on how nanotechnology-based advancements lead to novel drug delivery and treatment solutions.

It is a valuable research resource that will help both practicing medics and researchers in pharmaceutical science and nanomedicine learn more about how nanotechnology improves treatments.

KEY FEATURES

- Theoretical aspects of the subject have been written in the elementary language.
- Sightsees how nanotechnology is being used to create more efficient drug delivery systems.
- Deliberates which nanomaterials make the best drug carriers.
- Evaluates the opportunities and challenges of nanotechnology-based drug delivery systems.

Readership targets biomaterials scientists, pharmaceutical scientists, toxicologists, biomedical engineers, medicinal chemists, and postgraduate students specializing in nanomedicine, bio nanomaterials, and nanotechnology applications in healthcare.

Massive efforts have been made to keep this book error free, despite that, if any error or whatsoever is skipped in the book, it is purely incidental; we apologize for the same. Please write to us about that so that it can be corrected in the future edition of the book.

In the end, we would like to wish the best of luck to our readers!

1 Introduction

In recent times, nanotechnology has become a popular term representing the main efforts of the current science and technology. According to National Nanotechnology Initiative (NNI), nanoparticles are defined as structures of sizes ranging from 1 to 100 nm in at least one dimension, and nanotechnology is defined as "Science, engineering, and technology conducted at the nanoscale, ranging from 1 to 100 nanometres."

One of the significant areas of nanotechnology is "nanomedicine," which, according to the National Institute of Health (NIH) Nanomedicine Roadmap Initiative, refers to highly specific medical intervention for diagnosis, prevention, and treatment of diseases at the molecular scale.

These nanomaterials have been reported to show promising potential in key industries, specifically in nanomedicine, pharmacology, and the biomedical field which influences the frontiers of nanomedicine starting from biosensors, microfluidics, drug delivery, and microarray analysis to tissue engineering.

Nanosized materials that possess the capability to carry a drug/multiple drugs and/or imaging agent are called nanocarriers. The involvement of nanocarriers as drug delivery vehicles has various merits over free drug administration. Cells uptake the nanoparticles with optimized physicochemical and biological properties more easily compared with larger molecules, thus they can be used as drug delivery tools for various bioactive compounds. The high surface area to volume ratio makes the nanocarriers suitable to carry a large number of ligands on their surface for targeting. Nanocarriers increase local drug concentration by encapsulating the drug and liberating it in a controlled manner to the target cells and tissues.

Engineered nanomaterials (ENMs), with a size of 100 nm or less, are synthesized from several types of nanomaterials. These ENMs offer great opportunities to nanomedicine, and they have been increasingly commercialized in several industries and can be engineered at nanoscale to tune the delivery and releasing efficiency (Figure 1.1).

Particles size in nanoscale exhibits unique structural, chemical, mechanical, magnetic, electrical, and biological properties. Nanostructures are utilized as delivery agents either by encapsulating drugs or by attaching therapeutic drugs and delivering them to target tissues more precisely with an organized release. These nanostructures remain in the blood circulatory system for a prolonged period and enable the release of amalgamated drugs as per the indicated dose. Thus, they root for less plasma fluctuations with reduced adverse effects. Being nanosized, these structures breach the tissue system and assist easy uptake of the drug by cells, thus permitting an efficient drug delivery and ensuring action at the targeted site. The uptake of nanostructures by cells is much higher than that of large particles with sizes ranging between 1 and 10 µm. Hence, they directly interact to treat the diseased cells with enhanced efficiency and reduced or negligible side effects.

DOI: 10.1201/9781003252122-1

1

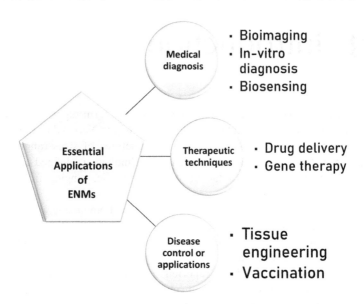

FIGURE 1.1   Essential applications of ENMs.

Among all other significant applications of ENMs, one of them is the specialized drug delivery in deploying liposomes to nanoshells and transdermal patches. At the same time, the development of biocompatible nanomaterial prosthetic implants and the use of metal-enclosing functionalized nanoparticles have shown high localization, patient-specific functionalities in the bioimaging, and treatment of various cancers. By integrating ENMs usage to artificial intelligence technologies, ENMs can realize the development of internet-linked diagnostic devices (e.g., "doctor-on-a-chip" diagnostic tools).

2 Nano-Based Drug Delivery System

2.1 INTRODUCTION

The conservative use of drugs presents challenging problems in the treatment of many diseases in terms of therapeutic effectiveness, poor biodistribution, stability, solubility and absorption by the intestine, lack of selectivity, side effects, and instabilities in plasma concentration. Drug delivery systems (DDSs) have been designed to overcome these limitations as well as drawbacks. DDS provides specific targeting of drug and its delivery, using lower doses of drug minimizes undesirable side effects and protects the drug from degradation. Recent progress in nanotechnology has indicated that nanoparticles (ranging in size from 1 to 1,000 nm) can be successfully used as drug carriers with adjusted physicochemical and biological properties, such as small size, increased drug accumulation, therapeutic effects, ability to cross the tissue barrier, controlled drug release, etc. Based on shape, nanoparticles can be of 0D, 1D, 2D, or 3D structure types, and depending on their source/type of materials, they can be separated into different categories such as carbon-based, metal-based, semiconductor-based, ceramic-based, polymeric-based, and lipid-based nanoparticles.

The framework of these nanoparticles can be analyzed using polarized optical microscopy (POM), Brunauer–Emmett–Teller (BET), scanning electron microscopy (SEM), X-ray diffraction (XRD), transmission electron microscopy (TEM), atomic force microscopy (AFM), Raman spectroscopy, X-ray photoelectron spectroscopy (XPS), infrared (IR), and Zeta size analyzer.

The use of nanoparticles as drug carriers plays a vital role in eradicating the challenging problems associated with conventional drugs used for the treatment of many chronic diseases such as hypertension, cancer, asthma, human immunodeficiency virus (HIV), and diabetes.

Polymeric-based nanocarriers, dendrimers, polymeric micelles, liposomes, solid lipids nanoparticles (SLNs), metallic nanoparticles (magnetic, gold), carbon nanotubes, nanospheres, nanocapsules, and nanogels are examples of nano-based drug delivery systems that are currently under research and development. Food and Drug Administration (FDA) had approved the clinical use of some of them, especially in cancer treatment (Figure 2.1).

DOI: 10.1201/9781003252122-2

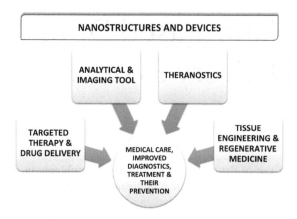

FIGURE 2.1   Nanotechnology deployed in various biomedical applications.

2.2 THERANOSTICS

Theranostic Nanoparticles (NPs) can be used for custom-made nanomedicine-based therapies. NPs are frequently conjugated with suitable targeting ligands on the surface of the particles. Multifunctional NPs can be established by integrating various functional materials, and this enables multimodal imaging and therapy simultaneously, also known as *theranostic*. Theranostic involves the administration of a diagnosis agent and is referred to as a combination of diagnosis and therapy using the same agent. Theranostic NPs can help in the diagnosis of the disease, reporting the location, identifying the stage of the disease, and providing information about the treatment response. Besides, such nanoparticles can carry a therapeutic agent for the tumor, which can provide the essential concentrations of the therapeutic agent via molecular and/or external stimuli.

- **Multimodality Imaging:** Superparamagnetic Iron Oxide Nanoparticles (SPIONs), (Feraheme, FH) and Zirconium [^{89}Zr] were used as a nanoplatform for photoemission tomography (PET) and magnetic resonance imaging (MRI). PET-MRI integrates the excellent sensitivity of PET with the spatial resolution and contrast of soft tissue by MRI. FH radiolabeled with PET tracer can take advantage of highly sensitive bright signals from PET. It can identify the presence of FH in regions where the MRI contrast is too low or noisy. Experimental data have shown that FH is a very suitable SPION for chelate-free labeling of PET tracers, and it can be used in hybrid PET-MRI.
- **Image-Guided Therapy:** A semiconducting plasmonic nanovesicle was proposed that consisted of semiconducting polyperylene diimide (PPDI) and polyethylene glycol (PEG) tethered to gold NPs (Au-PPDI/PEG). The complex was highly localized and possesses a strong electromagnetic field between the adjacent gold NPs in the vesicular shell. The electromagnetic field enhanced the light absorption efficiency of PPDI and generates a great

photothermal effect. It also provides a strong photoacoustic signal that can be used in photoacoustic imaging (PAI). Overall, the complex has a high potential suitable for a theranostic agent.

- **Combination Therapy:** It provides treatment for several malignancies to progress clinical outcomes. Several NPs are used in combination therapy such as (i) Liposomes which are one of the most recognized drug delivery vehicles, with many clinical products, (ii) Polymeric NPs which have high thermodynamic and kinetic properties used in site-specific delivery of the anticancer drug to tumors, (iii) Metallic NPs, dendrimers, nanodiamonds, carbon NPs, and carbon nanotubes (CNTs) which are the other ones used in combination therapy. A mesoporous NP-based drug delivery system has been introduced to be used for real-time imaging in photothermal/photodynamic therapy and nanozyme oxidative therapy.

2.3   TARGETED THERAPY AND DRUG DELIVERY

Traditionally, non-specific drug administration caused the distribution of drugs throughout the body, with the very little amount of drug reaching the desired physiological target tissue or cell type which results in lower drug efficacy and unwanted side effects on other parts of the body. Delivering drugs in such a way that their concentration is increased in the target tissue and reduced in healthy tissues, thus increasing efficacy and lowering side effects, can be accomplished through targeted drug delivery. Targeted drug delivery can be used in the treatment of various physiological disorders like diabetes and cardiovascular diseases, but it finds its most promising application in the area of cancer treatment.

The advantages of nanocarriers over free drug through targeted delivery are the following:

1. Protection of drug from early degradation
2. Increased time in blood circulation
3. Increased shelf life
4. Superior absorption of drugs by the target tissue
5. Organized release of drug in target cells/tissues
6. Improved intracellular penetration

For an effective drug delivery to the target, there are four conditions required, which include holding drug-carrying vehicles in the system, evading the immune system, reaching the target, and releasing the drug.

2.4   ANALYTICAL AND IMAGING TOOL

Nanomaterials are frequently used in biomedical imaging and cancer therapy. They make an excellent drug carrier, photothermal agents, imaging contrast agents due to their high sensitivity, small size, and composition, photoacoustic agents, and radiation dose enhancers, among their other applications. The medical imaging modalities comprise ultrasound, optical imaging, MRI, computed tomography,

PET, single-photon emission computerized tomography, and photoacoustic imaging. Various cancer therapeutic methods are also included such as photothermal therapy, photodynamic therapy, chemotherapy, and immunotherapy. Unique and intrinsic features of nanoparticles, i.e., its magnetic or optical properties, make their application ideal for various imaging modalities. However, no single molecular imaging modality can offer all the required data, fully characterizing the properties of an administered agent. Each imaging modality has a major shortcoming, such as MRI has high resolution but low sensitivity, optical techniques have restricted tissue penetration, and radioisotope imaging techniques have relatively poor resolution but high sensitivity. Multiple imaging techniques are integrated to enable these applications to counterpart one another, and a multimodal imaging agent becomes the key to augment those imaging systems. Medical imaging has improved significantly in recent decades and allows deciphering anatomical information via different modalities precisely. The contribution of NPs in medical imaging is discussed below:

1. **Magnetic Resonance Imaging:** MRI is a non-invasive medical imaging technique used in radiology to form pictures of the anatomy and the physiological processes of the body. MRI scanners involve the use of strong magnetic fields and gradients, and radio waves to generate images of the organs in the body.

2. **Computed Tomography (CT):** CT works by making use of an X-ray source and a detector array to form images. It can yield an image with high spatial and temporal resolution. It can provide 3D anatomical information of specific tissues and organs, but it lacks sensitivity toward contrast agents; in contrast, other modalities such as MRI shines utilize gold nanoparticles that possess antique X-ray attenuation properties as well as easy surface modification. AuNPs can be made functional with glucosamine to act as an effective contrast agent. Gold nanoparticles have a high X-ray absorption coefficient, and they can specifically image tumors using CT with an enhanced permeability and retention (EPR) effect. Iodine-based (^{131}I) polymer iodine NP contrast agents were hosted for high vascular contrast and tumor loading. They are economic and their organic structure provides biodegradation and clearance compared to other metal NPs. They are also very small (~20 nm) in size, which provides better tumor penetration compared to larger NPs. The contrast agents have a long blood half-life (40 h) that provides better tumor uptake and clearance from the liver when compared to AuNPs. Hydrophobic Bismuth (Bi_2S_3) NPs and quantum dots could be used as a contrast enhancer for collective CT/fluorescence imaging.

3. **Positron Emission Tomography (PET):** PET is a nuclear medicine imaging technique. Radiotracers are used to produce images of radionuclide distribution. These tracers can provide information on biological pathways through a non-invasive method.

4. **Single-Photon Emission Computerized Tomography (SPECT):** SPECT is a nuclear imaging technique that uses gamma rays to assess biochemical changes and the level of the molecular target within a living subject.

TABLE 2.1

The Use of Nanoparticles in Different Imaging Techniques (for Detailed Study Refer to Chapter 6)

	Imaging Techniques	Nanoparticles Involved
1	Magnetic resonance imaging	Gadolinium (Gd), SPIONs, carbon, manganese (Mn), silicon, peptide
2	Computed tomography	Gold nanoparticles, iodine, bismuth
3	Positron emission tomography	Gold nanoparticles, copper, other nanoparticles
4	Single photon emission computerized tomography	Gold nanoparticles, technetium
5	Optical imaging	Fluorescent NPs, quantum dots, gold nanoparticles, persistent luminescence NPs
6	Ultrasound	Chitosan
7	Photoacoustic imaging	Gold nanoparticles, carbon nanotube, fluorescent NPs

5. **Optical Imaging:** Non-invasive optical imaging can screen various classes of structures that are involved in autophagy at both macroscopic and microscopic levels. Optical imaging is involved in chemiluminescence, fluorescence, and Raman imaging, which can obtain non-invasive 2-dimensional or multidimensional image data at the macro- and micro-scale. Fluorescence imaging provides intuitive results, takes less time, and can more easily be interpreted compared to other methods. That is why it is usually preferred by researchers and is used in a biomedical imaging application.

6. **Ultrasound:** Ultrasound is also a non-invasive imaging technique that can evaluate morphology, orientation, internal structure, and margins of the lesion from multiple planes with a high resolution predominantly in both fatty breast and dense glandular structures. Ultrasound-guided drug delivery using nanobubbles (NBs) has evolved into a promising strategy in recent years. NBs usually comprise gas cores and stabilized shells. They can easily cross the capillary wall, and they have been used in many targeted therapies for cancer treatment such as 5-fluorouracil loaded NBs for hepatocellular carcinoma.

7. **Photoacoustic Imaging (PAI):** PAI is based on the photoacoustic effect. It recreates images from captured ultrasound signals generated from the materials that thermally expand by the laser pulse. It is frequently referred to as optoacoustic imaging. It is a cost-effective modality that can provide regional imaging of blood vessels. It has high spatial and temporal resolution with clinically agreed imaging depth (Table 2.1).

2.5 TISSUE ENGINEERING AND REGENERATIVE MEDICINE

Tissue engineering (TE) is an interdisciplinary field integrating engineering, material science, and medical biology that aims to develop biological alternatives for repairing, replacing, retaining, or enhancing tissue and organ-level functions.

TE is the study of the progression of new tissues and organs, starting from a base of cells and scaffolds. These scaffolds are 3D structures in which the cells grow, proliferate, and differentiate into various cell types. Growth factors are introduced into these scaffolds to direct the cell behavior toward any desired process where the subsequent goal is to produce fully functional organs or tissues that are capable of growth and regeneration and are suitable for implantation. Despite such promises, current TE methods face obstacles including a lack of appropriate biomaterials, ineffective cell growth, and a lack of techniques for seizing appropriate physiological architectures as well as imbalanced and inadequate production of growth factors to stimulate the cell communication and proper response. Besides, the inability to control cellular functions and their various properties (biological, mechanical, electrochemical, and others) and issues of biomolecular detection and biosensors, all add up to the current limitations in this field.

The surface conjugation and conducting properties of gold NPs (AuNPs), the antimicrobial properties of silver and other metallic nanoparticles and metal oxides, the fluorescence properties of quantum dots, and the unique electromechanical features of CNTs have made them beneficial in numerous TE applications. Additionally, magnetic nanoparticles have also been applied in the research of cell mechanic transduction, gene delivery, controlling cell patterning, and construction of complex 3D tissues.

TE can significantly enhance the biological, mechanical, as well as electrical properties of scaffolds which can serve various functions depending on the applications as described in the following points:

- **Biological Property Enhancement:** Increased cell proliferation rates: nanoparticles in particular, namely of two types, AuNPs and titanium dioxide (TiO_2) nanoparticles, have been used to boost cell proliferation rates for regeneration of bone and cardiac tissue, respectively. AuNPs have shown superior biocompatibility and the ability for surface modification which have resulted in exciting biomedical applications.
- **Enhancement of Mechanical Properties:** Nanoparticles-implanted nanocomposite polymers in either forms, hydrogels and electrospun fibers, have displayed superior mechanical properties for TE applications as compared to scaffolds without nanoparticle reinforcements. For example, a TiO_2-impregnated biodegradable patch presented a higher tensile strength in underpinning the scar after myocardial infarction.
- **For Skin TE:** 3D nanocomposite scaffolds were prepared using a mixture of type I collagen and polyvinylpyrrolidone (PVP)-coated titanium dioxide (TiO_2) nanoparticles. Hydrogen bonds were formed in this blend between collagen, PVP, and TiO_2, which improves the ultimate tensile strength of these scaffolds.
- **Enhancement of Electrical Properties:** Gold nanowires have also been cast-off as conductive materials alongside scaffolds to enhance the electrical coupling between the cells. With time, cardiac muscle cells started developing within the 3D porous scaffolds and resulted in synapse formation.

- **Antibacterial Applications:** Silver nanoparticles are known to possess great antimicrobial effects, as well as wound healing capabilities. Antibacterial activity of poly 3-hydroxybutyrate-co-3-hydroxyvalerate (PHBV) nano-fibrous scaffolds containing silver has found that silver-containing PHBV nanofibrous scaffolds had high antibacterial properties and they demonstrated brilliant in vitro cell compatibility. This shows that PHBV nanofibrous scaffolds containing silver nanoparticles have visions to be used in joint arthroplasty, and thus, should be further studied. Another study dealing with the categorization and antimicrobial activity of a nano silver-based biocomposite skeleton for bone TE suggested that biocomposite scaffolds containing nanosilver own the capability to regulate bacterial infection during reconstructive bone surgery and that the presence of Ag NPs in the scaffolds acted as an affixed coating for protection against infection, sepsis, and malfunctioning of implants.
- **Gene Delivery:** For effective gene therapy applications, it is vital to construct a suitable vector system with properties such as a high gene transfection efficiency, low cytotoxicity, and high specificity to unhealthy cells.
- **Constructing 3D Tissues:** Skin keratinocyte sheets consisting of five or more cellular layers were constructed, which were sufficiently strong for improvement, and the sheets comprised of undifferentiated keratinocytes that may be more effective in wound healing.

3 Drug Designing and Drug Delivery

3.1 INTRODUCTION

Nanomedicine is the medical sector that uses nanotechnology science to treat various diseases using nanoscale materials such as biocompatible nanoparticles and nanorobots for diagnostics, delivery, sensory, or performance purposes in a living organism. Delivery means the ability to convey an agent to a particular targeted place in the body from outside the body (or biological system). The delivery may rest on the size, shape, surface chemistry, rigidity, and chemical composition of the distributing vehicles, but the ideal design is still indefinite to achieve a given biological goal. During the journey from site to destination, biological systems with which nanoparticles engage represent barriers to the delivery process. Compared to bigger equivalents that can help medication delivery systems, nanomaterials display distinct chemical and physical characteristics and biological efficacy. The high surface-to-volume relationship, chemical and geometric tunability of nanoparticles, and their ability to interact with biomolecules are significant benefits of promoting absorption through the cell membranes. The vast area is also associated with medicine and tiny molecules for targeted and controlled releases such as ligands or antibodies.

3.1.1 JOURNEY OF NANOPARTICLE

Nanoparticular–biological (nano–bio) interactions are the relationship between the designed nanomaterial and the biological system. Proteins get adsorbed on the surface of the nanoparticle immediately and create a protein corona when acquainted with nanoparticles. This protein corona profile of nanoparticle first interacts with the nanoparticle's physical and chemical features, such as the height, shape, and surface load, and relies on biological molecule and liquid (such as blood, cerebrospinal fluid, and saliva). It establishes a novel interface between nanoparticles and cells or tissues, affecting nanoparticles' absorption, biodistribution, and immune response. The formed protein corona may change the in vivo trajectory of the nanoparticle. The targeting effect of designed ligands on nanoparticles surface can also be concealed by formed protein corona. Most blood-circulating nanoparticles are generally eliminated by the liver and spleen of the reticuloendothelial system (RES). The purpose of such organs is to filter blood and remove it from the circulation of biological waste and foreign particles. The organ is a significant obstacle in administering intravenous nanoparticles such as quantum dots, micelles, gold nanoparticles, and liposomes.

DOI: 10.1201/9781003252122-3

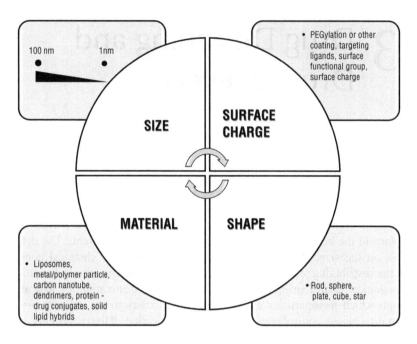

FIGURE 3.1 Illustration of biophysiochemical properties of explored nanoparticle as a carrier in drug delivery.

The liver can sequestrate the majority of injected nanoparticles and store non-degradable nanoparticles for months after administration. Kupffer cells are the main source of sequestration. The phagocytic immune cells that line the interior of sinusoids of the liver can catch nanoparticles as they circulate. However, avoidance of RES is crucial for enhancing the efficacy of administration of intravenous nanoparticles to destinations outside RES. Kidneys can extricate nanoparticles below 6 nm in size, and dendritic cells can sequestrate nanoparticles that are intradermally administered. The physiology of the vessel determines the transport of nanoparticles through the blood vessel. The surface charge and form of nanoparticles, like shape and size, may significantly impact the clearance of the nanoparticles by the kidneys. Solid tumor vessels employ both an active and a passive method of transport to transfer nanoparticles (Figure 3.1).

The physicochemical characteristics of the nanoparticle, such as size, surface chemistry, and charge, should be tailored to extravasate at the target tissue through blood arteries. Through the tissue stroma, the nanoparticles inside the target tissue should pass to reach the target cells. Extracellular matrix (ECM) and connective tissue cells, such as fibroblast, pericyte, and supportive tissue-specific cells, are present in the tissue stroma. Nanoparticles can be trapped in extracellular matrix proteins before they can get to their destination. The ECM's composition varies across the tissue and it is subject to significant liver fibrosis or cancer conditions changes. Some ECM elements, including collagen, fibrinogen, and hyaluronic acid, may sterically impede the dissemination of nanoparticles. Stromal off-target cells can trap nanoparticles before they reach the target type. Nanoparticles should traverse through tissue stroma and escape ECM or off-target cell sequestration or destruction to reach their target.

3.2 DRUG DEVELOPMENT

Creating novel medication systems takes time; the fundamental research and development process takes roughly seven years before supporting preclinical animal research. Nanoparticle delivery focuses on medication effectiveness maximization and cytotoxicity minimization (Figure 3.2).

The following variables are addressed in order to refine nanoparticles characteristics for efficient drug delivery:

- More ligand binding to the surface is achievable by changing the surface area to the volume proportion of nanoparticles. Increased effectiveness of ligand binding would result in lower doses and reduction in toxicity of nanoparticles. Reduction in dose frequency or dosage also reduces the mass of nanoparticles per drug mass, increasing efficiency.
- Another significant design feature is the surface functionalization of nanoparticles and it frequently involves the bioconjugation or passive absorption of molecules on the surface of the nanoparticles. More significant potential and lower toxicity are achieved by working with nanoparticles

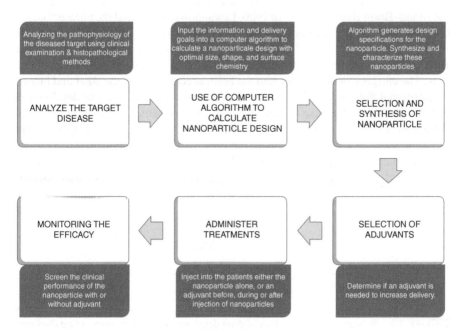

FIGURE 3.2   A coherent approach for designing and testing of nanoformulations for drug delivery (Poon et al., 2020).

and ligands to improve drug binding, inhibit immune response, or regulate release capability. Effectiveness is enhanced by delivering more medicine to the target location and limiting the body's harmful side effects. Depending upon the intended environment or desired impact, the composition of nanoparticles can be chosen. For instance, following the delivery of liposome-based nanoparticles, the danger of accumulation and toxicity may be reduced biologically after the release of therapeutic cargo is reduced. Metal nanoparticles, such as gold nanoparticles, have optical properties, which provide less invasive imaging techniques. In addition, nanoparticles can be used directly for tumor treatment to respond photothermally to optical stimulation (Figure 3.3).

For further study on nanoparticle supply systems, the National Institute of Biomedical Imaging and Bioengineering has published the following prospects:

1. Blood–brain barrier (BBB) crossing in brain illnesses and disorders;
2. focused enhancement of intracellular delivery to guarantee the suitable structures within the cells is achieved;
3. an amalgamation of diagnostics and therapy.

3.2.1 Drug delivery via blood–brain barrier

The central nervous system (CNS) has one of the strongest endothelial systems, i.e., the Blood–Brain Barrier (BBB). In 1900, Lewandowsky invented the phrase "blood–brain barrier" (BBB). The human brain has around hundred billion endothelial capillaries with a distribution of 650 km, covering a total area of roughly 20 m^2. The BBB contains endothelial cells, astrocytes, pericytes, microglial neurons, and neurons. The entrance of substances into the brain is controlled by the BBB and blood–cerebrospinal fluid barrier. It is regarded as the barrier to the effective development of CNS medicines. Because of their difficulty in penetrating the BBB, most neuro-therapeutic chemicals never reach the market. The BBB's remarkable selectivity owes to the presence of endothelial cells in the brain. Adherens junctions (AJs) between endothelial cells and tight junctions (TJs) function as the physical barrier. This small interconnect network provides BBB with greater than 1500 Ωm^2 of trans-electric

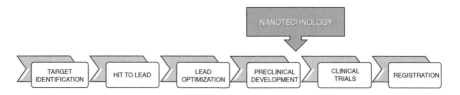

FIGURE 3.3 Schematic representation of drug development process representing the interface between medicinal chemistry and nanotechnology (Sanna and Sechi, 2020).

resistance. The functions of the immunological barrier are served by microglia, perivascular macrophages, and mast cells. The internal and external enzymes in the endothelial cells function as metabolic barriers to the organelle-specific targeting of lipophilic substances.

3.2.2 ORGANELLE-SPECIFIC TARGETING

Ultimate efficiency of the carrier in delivering its cargo to the intracellular activity location depends on the efficiency of any designed nano item. Successfully targeted and internalized carriers bearing oligonucleotide as a payload must pass the nuclear membrane to be efficacious. However, the oligonucleotides may be destroyed under severe lysosomal conditions unless they escape from the endosome. This underlines that techniques are needed to guide designed nanoparticles to particular subcellular cells. Operative organelle targeting tools and concepts such as the target delivery to nucleus, cytosol, mitochondria, peroxisomes, and endosomes/lysosomes are being developed.

3.3 DESIGNING NANOPARTICLES FOR THERAPEUTICS

The technique of providing suitable amounts of treatment agents to the afflicted area of the body is the targeted therapy in illness treatment over a lengthy duration. To this end, the evolution of more safe and efficient therapeutic nanoparticles is essential and one of the nanomedicine's ultimate objectives. They are prone to aggregation and protein opsonization as soon as nanoparticles enter the circulation (protein binding to nanoparticle surface as a tag for immune system recognition). The opsonized nanoparticles can be removed from the circulation by phagocytosis or filtration in the liver, spleen, and kidney. This quick and non-specific immune clearance reduces retention time and hence lowers bioavailability (Yetisgin et al., 2020).

In the cells, most nanoparticles are absorbed through endocytosis by clathrin or caveolae-related mechanisms. Due to the internalization of nanoparticles by target cells, the form is also vital for biodistribution. For example, cationic nanoparticles in rod form have more straightforward endosomal goals than cationic nanoparticles in other forms, which may lead immune system cells to mistake these nanoparticles for rod-shaped bacteria.

Perceptions on the Design of Nanoparticle Carriers: A poly metro conjugated synthesis in the 1950s may be the earliest attempt to develop a therapy based on nanoparticles. In the past nanoparticle, carriers have been made and tested with a more extensive range of materials, including protein, polysaccharides, synthetic polymers, metals, and several other organic/inorganic substances; in order to accomplish the site-expected release of the drugs with optimum therapeutic rates and dosing records, the composition, size, shape, surface characteristics, biocompatibility, and degradation profile should be carefully developed and optimized as an essential requirement for drug delivery carriers (Table 3.1).

TABLE 3.1
Factors Influencing the Biodistribution of Drug-Laden Nanocarriers

Attributes	Description
Natural/synthetic constituents	By established routes, a biological system may readily identify and metabolically digest naturally occurring beneficial compounds, whereas the synthetic ones can lead to toxicity, persistent inflammation, and clearance problems. Nevertheless, a natural approach is limiting due to the absence of special optical/electric/magnetic characteristics, lot-to-lot variability, immunogenicity, insufficient biomechanical qualities, and structural complexity. Currently, nanoparticles based on synthetic materials are a dominant feeder because they enable fine control of the formulation's physicochemical characteristics. Nanoparticles should be stable, physiologically inert, and nontoxic to deliver anticancer to the tumor locations in vivo. At the same time, they must stay in the bloodstream long enough to reach the target site and go through the target site several times. Therefore, the surface charges and hydrophobicity of nanoparticles can be adapted and improved for half-life with the use of synthetic materials to increase their circulation. Moreover, its surface functionality may be designed easily to optimize its affinity to the target receptors (Sun et al., 2014)
Size and shape	The main features are particle sizes and size distribution because nanomaterials' chemical and physical characteristics are determined by these. In vivo dispersion, biological destiny, toxicity, and these nanomaterials' ability for drug supplies are determined by the hydrodynamic and size distribution. To handle the loading, release, and stability of drugs, nanomaterials are beneficial over microparticles, and since they are tiny and highly mobile, they may be used more efficiently for more cellular and intracellular objectives. By changing zeta, potential attachment or adsorption of a charged molecule can be determined on the surface of the nanoparticle (Prabhakar and Banerjee, 2020)
Surface properties • Surface charges	Surface charge is usually expressed and measured in terms of the nanomaterials' zeta potential, which reflects the electrical potential of particles influenced by their composition and the medium in which it is dispersed. Zeta potential having a value of ± 30 mV has been reported to be stable in suspension, leading to prevention of particle aggregation. The surface charge of nanomaterials is crucial for drug loading. Drugs can be loaded via several processes such as covalent conjugation, hydrophobic interaction, charge–charge interaction, or encapsulation. Loading of molecules depends on the nature of the drug and the nature of the target molecule, which also alters the surface charge. By changing zeta, potential attachment or adsorption of a charged molecule can be determined on the surface of the nanoparticle (Jahan et al., 2017)
• PEGylation	Brush-like PEG coatings decrease phagocytosis and complement activation; those with a mushroom like shape complement potent phagocytosis activators. PEGylation is frequently used to preserve nanoparticles like liposomes, polymer nanoparticles, and micelles from premature clearance during circulation since the actual usage of PEG increases the circulatory half-life of a protein. The PEG chains form a hydrated shell to avoid opsonization and subsequent phagocytosis in the nanoparticles. This shell can nevertheless interfere with the interactions between a nanoparticle and the target cell (Sun et al., 2014)

(Continued)

TABLE 3.1 (*Continued*)
Factors Influencing the Biodistribution of Drug-Laden Nanocarriers

Attributes	Description
• Polysaccharides • Conjugation with targeting ligands	*Polysaccharides* have been widely employed for the supply of drugs and tissue engineering due to their high biocompatibility. As a result, several polysaccharides such as dextran and heparin have been characterized as stalking materials due to their capacity to prevent supplementary system and opsonization. Some investigations have revealed some ligand activities in their polysaccharides, such as chitosan and hyaluronic acid. Because of unique interactions with different receptors on the surface of the target cells, nanoparticles covered with these polysaccharides exhibit more effective cellular absorption than other nanoparticles
Drug loading	Drug loading is known as the incorporation of a drug into or on nanoparticles. A high medication loading capacity without aggregation should be an excellent nanoparticle delivery method. High load capacity for medicines helps decreasing the number of dosages or administration. Smooth and effective distribution of medicines requires dispersibility. Drug loading may be performed in a variety of ways. However, the efficiency of the drug loading and trapping may depend on nanoparticles, the dispersion medium, size and composition of nanomaterials, drug molecules, drug molecular weight and solubility, interaction with drug nanomaterials and surfaces functional (i.e., carboxylic, amine, and ester) on the nanomaterials (Sun et al., 2014)

3.4   DELIVERY AND RELEASE MECHANISM

An effective targeted and controlled release of the drug should have an optimal medication delivery mechanism. Passive and active targeting are the two primary targeting methods. Passive targeting hinges on the improperly molded blood arteries due to tumors, encouraging hefty macromolecules and nanoparticles accretion. This alleged enhanced permeability and retention (EPR) effect allows the pharmaceutical carrier to be precisely delivered to the tumor cells. As per its name, active targeting is significantly better and is done by using interactions between the receiver and the ligand at the cell membrane surface. Many approaches may be used to develop controlled medication release systems. Rate-programmed drug delivery systems are adapted to the membrane distribution of active substances (Bennet and Kim, 2013). The activation-modulated drug delivery is another delivery method where environmental stimuli cause the release. The stimuli can be external, such as photoactivation, electromagnetic and biological activities like pH, temperature, and osmotic pressure, which can significantly differ in the whole body.

Drugs with extremely poor solubility have several problems administering biopharmaceuticals, including restricted bio accessibility following oral intake, less spreading ability into the outer membrane, and additional intravenous intakes. However, the use of nanotechnology techniques in the medication delivery mechanism might circumvent all these constraints. Nano-design has been well researched and is by far the most sophisticated nanoparticles technology in terms of its future benefits, such as the possibility of modifying characteristics like solubility, profile release, diffusion, bioavailability, and immunogenicity. Therefore, this can enhance and create comfortable management methods, less toxicity, less adverse effects, improved biodistribution, and longer pharmaceutical cycles (Patra et al., 2018). The tailored medicines are either targeted at a specific place or designed to regulate therapeutic liberation at a particular location. Their development consists of self-assemblies where spontaneously building pieces are generated in well-defined structures or patterns. They also need the mononuclear phagocyte system to overcome obstacles such as opsonization or sequestration (Blanco et al., 2015). Nanostructures distribute medicines in two ways: passive and self-delivery. The former involves medications primarily through the hydrophobic effect in the interior cavity of the structure. If the nanostructure components are directed at a particular spot, a low drug content contained in a hydrophobic environment frees the intending quantity of the drug. In this technique, the moment of release is critical since the medication does not reach the target location and disconnects from the carrier very fast; on the other hand, if it is released at the correct time from its nanostructure system, bioactivity and effectiveness will be lowered. The focus of medicinal products is another significant element that is classified into active and passive nanomaterials or nanoformulation systems for the delivery of medicines. Drives such as antibodies, peptides, and the medication delivery system are linked to the active targeting to attach them to the target location's receptor structures. The produced drug carriers circulate in passive targeting via the bloodstream and are pushed to the target location through affinity or binding conditions such as pH, temperature, molecular site, and form. The body's primary objectives are cell membrane receptors, cell membrane lipids, and cell antigens or proteins. Most medication delivery systems mediated by nanotechnology are currently focused on cancer and its treatment.

- Targeted Drug Delivery Methods
    i. **Passive Targeting:** Medication targeting is designated as a selective discharge into a particular organ, tissue, or cell at a physiological location that requires remarkable pharmacological influence. Active and passive processes are included with nanocarrier-driven cell targeting. When targeted passively, the medications can be supplied to the target organ based on pharmaceutical permanency in blood and preferential accumulation in the site of interest of the drug-laden nano supply system. The principal characteristic of tumor tissue is its out-of-order blood vessels, which enhances its vascular permeability (Chenthamara et al., 2019). This particular feature facilitates the transportation of macromolecules in tumor tissues. Maeda and other colleagues have also shown an increase in permeability and retention (EPR) impact on sites of infection or inflammation in which extra bradykinin is produced. Duration of retention periods is the primary distinction between the EPR effect caused by infections and the tumor effect. The swelling period is shorter for normal tissues, while the lymphatic drainage system is active in malignant tissues. This can disperse swelling after a few days. In cancer, increased permeability of the circulatory system leads to the tumor tissues having enough nutrition and oxygen for

rapid development. This particular pathophysiology and abnormality of tumor blood vessels is used to provide the tumor tissue with the medication molecules. Macromolecules more than 40 kDa will spread and become concentrated in tumor tissues from the tumor vasculature. This EPR effect-driven drug supply lacks normal tissues. This unique EPR effect characteristic of the tumor cells is thus considered a milestone in tumor-focused chemotherapy and it becomes a world view approach to anticancer development that is relentlessly encouraging. Therefore, it is now the gold standard in designing anticancer medication and cancer methods, including gene delivery, molecular imagery, antibody therapy, micelles, liposomes, and protein–polymer conjugates (Yin et al., 2014). PEG is the primary polymer for the modification of proteins in order to make pharmaceutical delivery more efficient. PEGylated L-asparaginase has been utilized as an acute phase-3 lymphoblastic leukemia (ALL) therapy owing to a circulatory life of 5.7 days for the human population compared to 1.2 days for the native enzyme (Patel et al., 2017). As anticancer medicines, already several protein–polymer conjugates are available. Blood plasma components might increase circulation time in some situations. Gradishar et al.'s research found a greater response in women with metastatic breast cancer than the usual paclitaxel formulation when nanometer-sized albumin-bound paclitaxel (ABI007) was given intravenously. Likewise, paclitaxel transport in endothelial cells increased four to five times compared to conventional paclitaxel by the nanodrug ABI007. Styrene-maleic anhydride-neocarzinostatin (SMANCS), the colony-stimulating factor PEG-granulocyte and PEG-L-asparaginase are now available on the market and are currently accessible online which are being used against hepatocellular carcinoma, acute lymphoblastic leukemia, and chemotherapy-associated neutropenia, respectively. Large solutes cannot be delivered via passive targeting, and therefore, the need of an alternative tactic has led to the development of active approaches (Figure 3.4).

ii. **Active Targeting:** Active targeting must be based on a particular location attached to the surface of the pharmaceutical carriers. It uses molecular recognition patterns such as ligand receptors and antigen antibodies to provide medication to a particular area (Figure 3.5). This powerful connection gives the delivery system additional specificity. The active method can also be achieved by handling physical stimuli (temperature, pH, and magnetism). The ligand that is linked to the nanoparticle's surface interacts with its receiver when actively aiming at the target site. The effectiveness of the targeting of medicines depends on the choice of the target movement, which should be numerous, strongly related to binding cell receptors, and appropriate for chemical conjugation modifications. Active tumor therapy targeting ligands include folate, aptamers, and short RNA or DNA oligonucleotides, which may fold up in multiple conformations and include binding of ligands, antibodies, and peptides. Active targeting offers reduced toxicity for healthy

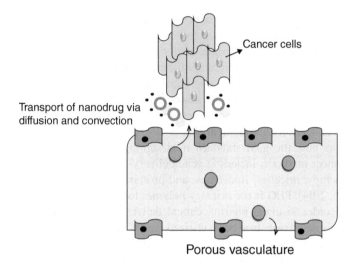

FIGURE 3.4 Drug delivery through passive targeting. Enhanced vascular permeability is characteristics of tumor cells along with the defective vascular anatomy that is exploited in passive targeting to improve the drug delivery by convection or passive diffusion in tumor cells.

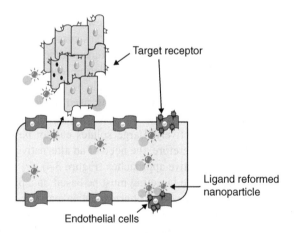

FIGURE 3.5 Drug delivery through active targeting. Targeting ligands are overexpressed in tumor cells, thus the desired nanoparticles are concocted to integrate ligand that will muddle to the target cells through ligand receptor collaboration.

tissues, as targeted ligands are overexpressed in the tumor tissue. Poor targeting and multidrug resistance (MDR) of tumors are two key barriers against carcinogenicity. The internalization of nanoparticles via receptor-mediated cell interactions is regarded as a successful technique in particular drug targeting. Several epithelial malignancies characterize the distinctive feature of folate receptor overexpression; they are therefore targeted for successful chemotherapy. Docetaxel (DTX) micelle is a ethoxy-poly(ethylene glycol)-folic acid (FA-PEG) micelle intended to exercise greater toxicity on Fr-positive MCF-7 cells (Shi et al., 2018). Increased targeting and binding on tumor cells using hyaluronic acid (HA) or its derivatives can transport numerous antitumor medicines, proteins, and nucleic acids and they are linked to overexpressed cell-surface receptors (Huang and Huang, 2018). Greater antitumor activity for squamous cell cancer cell lines OSC-19 and HN5 has been observed when HA–Paclitaxel conjugate (HA-PTX) upon bonding to CD44 receptor, thereby enhancing polymer–medicinal conjugate uptake. Matrix metalloproteinases (MMPs) are generally regarded to be cancer biomarkers, and a new approach to suppress the expression of MMPs is the development of a MMP-responsive system for the production of intelligent medication. The MMP substrates (Collagen, Gelatin, Fibrinogen, etc.) are developed into nanoparticles for such targeting systems. However, the therapeutic targeting or delivery of big proteins has severe constraints. In addition to being straightforward to integrate, the synthetic substrates (i.e., MMP-sensitive peptides) also offer selectivity and sensitivity. However, nanoparticles' MMP reactivity differs according to the choice of peptides. A self-assembling type copolymer glycol-phosphoethanolamine (PEG-pp-PE) was created to cure the use of both matrix metalloproteinase 2 (MMP2)-sensitive tumor targeting and P-glycoproteins (P-gp)-mediated drug efflux in order to treat drug-resistant malignancies (Chenthamara et al., 2019).

Nanoparticles can efficiently regulate the molecular size and surface characteristics of passive and active medication targeting with reduced adverse effects. The inclusion of nanoparticles protects the degradation of medicine. This method may be used for many routes such as oral, nasal, and parenteral. The drug will remain at a specific site in the right proportion for a prolonged time with less wastage and efficacy.

- In Vitro and In Vivo Delivery

Nanoparticles can increase medication concentrations in the tumor if enabled with either passive or active targeting capacity while lowering systemic toxicity in healthy tissues. Although the use of nanoparticles as medicinal products offers a lot of advantages, there are some problems that should be addressed throughout this process, including their volatility, low renal clearing, minimal build-up, blood circulation, poor absorption by malignant cells, and insufficient acceptance by cancer tissues. To counteract the mentioned complications, it is of great importance to have an inclusive understanding of the nanoparticles' responses by biological systems at cell, tissue, organ, and body levels (Table 3.2).

  - Comprehension of nanoparticles transport in vitro is a vital first step to their effective applications. On the one hand, before further in vivo testing at tissue, organ, and body levels, nanoparticles to act as drug carriers must first be assessed in vitro at the cellular level. On the other hand, one can begin to develop the characteristics of nanoparticles for optimal distribution in vivo and successful cancer treatment only

TABLE 3.2

The Foremost Phases Involved in the Delivery of a Nanoparticle

In Vitro	In Vivo
• Endocytosis	• The EPR effect and passive tumor targeting
• Intracellular transport	• Active tumor targeting
• Intracellular escape and degradation of nanoparticles	• Clearance by the MPS
• Multidrug resistance	• Renal clearance
	• Pharmacokinetics and biodistribution
	• Biocompatibility and biodegradation

with enough knowledge of nanoparticles–cells interactions. When a nanoparticle meets a cell, endocytosis will swiftly internalize it into the cell. Afterward, it will be transported to various organelles such as endosomes, lysosomes, mitochondria, endoplasmic reticulum (ER), and nucleus. The nanoparticles must be destroyed or demounted throughout the intracellular transport phase to ensure that their payload is released quickly.

• Although nanoparticles–cell interactions are mostly involved in in vitro drug delivery, this in vivo application highlights the way to move the carriers from their management location to the target lesion. Once the carriers are in, the target lesion must be reached and accumulated before any therapy is possible. As a result, several more concerns relating to nanoparticle transport, immune response, selectiveness, and efficacy must be addressed at organ and system level with regard to targeting, biodistribution, biodegradation, clearance, and toxicity. The nanoparticles that serve as carrier of a drug delivery system should ideally have the following attributes:

  – good focusing performance to guarantee a selective deposition of the drug into the target lesion while retaining low levels of healthy tissue/organ;
  – biocompatible and/or biodegradable materials only; however, all these conditions cannot be contented in authenticity (Sun et al., 2014).

3.5   CURRENT PROBLEMS AND CHALLENGES

In the present scenario, the following are the obstacles accompanying drug development and delivery which pharmaceutical companies are facing (Prabhakar and Banerjee, 2020):

• **Low Solubility:** The primary challenges with developing a particular formulation of the medicinal product are low aqueous solubility. The bioavailability of the drug is affected by poor solubility. It is, therefore, the main problem faced by scientists and industry for a new chemical entity.

- **Low Bioavailability:** The proportion of the accessible medication dosage for systemic circulation is bioavailability. It is one of medicine's most critical pharmacokinetic characteristics. The bioavailability of medication is 100% when administered intravenously, whereas its bioavailability stands compact by other routes (like orally) because of inadequate absorption. The bioavailability of a medication other than intravenously thus must be addressed during the administration.
- **Low Efficacy:** The most significant reaction obtained from an applied dosage of medication is low efficacy. The medication must provide high-affinity results in tight bindings to the target to be a highly efficient drug. This association is called drug molecule affinity. If the drug's affinity to the target molecule is poor, the maximal response will be diminished. Low effectiveness is one of the main difficulties in the treatment of serious illnesses related to the medication molecule.
- **Fast Excretion:** Removing the medication from the body by excretory organisms such as kidneys is called excretion or elimination. The drug molecule is quickly eradicated because the desired amount of drug molecule does not reach the target organs.
- **Fraction of Drug Required Zone Does Not Persist:** In some parts of an organ, the concentration of a drug in a certain quantity is required as high as that seen in normal cells for optimal therapy. The medication must concentrate on the tumor cell concentration. The lack of optimal drug accumulation with chemotherapy for cancer treatment is related to chemotherapeutic agents.

3.6   CONCLUSION

For the delivery of drugs, the formulation of nanoparticles (NPs) provides several benefits. Scientists may change NP formulations for various substances, depending on individual needs and interests. The use of NPs in development makes them excellent for application in several research fields. NPs offer a wide range of bio benefits: Drugs are protected against impairment and oxidation and those are used as a medication stabilizer, tissue targeting, and propagation aids. Surface alterations' variations for NPs provide flexibility in drug design and optional changes based on the particular research demands. NPs can enhance a range of medicines, pharmacokinetic and pharmacodynamic characteristics, minimize toxicity, and raise the criteria for medication safety. In the field of novel medication development, NP formulations offer a very workable option. Many of today's appropriate medications have been demonstrated to function well to reduce serious adverse effects. NPs are an effective alternative to side effects, risk reduction, and overall patient safety and quality of life in novel medicine development.

REFERENCES

Bennet, D,. & Kim, S. (2013). A transdermal delivery system to enhance quercetin nanoparticle permeability. *Journal of Biomaterials Science, Polymer Edition*, 24(2), 185–209.

Blanco, E., Shen, H., & Ferrari, M. (2015). Principles of nanoparticle design for overcoming biological barriers to drug delivery. *Nature Biotechnology*, 33, 941.

Chenthamara, D., Subramaniam, S., Ramakrishnan, S.G., Krishnaswamy, S.G., Essa, M.M., Lin, F.H., & Qoronfleh, M.W. (2019). Therapeutic efficacy of nanoparticles and routes of administration. *Biomaterials Research*, 23, 20. https://doi.org/10.1186/s40824-019-0166-x.

Gradishar, W.J., Tjulandin, S., Davidson, N., Shaw, H., Desai, N., Bhar, P., Hawkins, M., & O'Shaughnessy, J. (2005). Phase III trial of nanoparticle albumin-bound paclitaxel compared with polyethylated castor oil-based paclitaxel in women with breast cancer. *Journal of Clinical Oncology*, 23(31), 7794–7803.

Huang, G., & Huang, H. (2018). Hyaluronic acid-based biopharmaceutical delivery and tumor-targeted drug delivery system. *Journal of Controlled Release,* 278, 122–126.

Jahan, S.T., Sadat, S.M.A., Walliser, M., & Haddadi, A. (2017). Targeted therapeutic nanoparticles: An immense promise to fight against cancer. *Journal of Drug Delivery*, 2017, (iv), 1–24.

Maeda, H., Wu, J., Sawa, T., Matsumura, Y., & Hori, K. (2000). Tumor vascular permeability and the EPR effect in macromolecular therapeutics: a review. *Journal of Controlled Release*, 65(1–2), 271–284.

Mitchell, M.J., Billingsley, M.M., Haley, R.M., Wechsler, M.E., Peppas, N.A., & Langer, R. (2021). Engineering precision nanoparticles for drug delivery. *Nature Reviews Drug Discovery*, 20, 101–124. https://doi.org/10.1038/s41573-020-0090-8.

Patel, B., Kirkwood, A.A., Dey, A., Marks, D.I., McMillan, A.K., Menne, T.F., Micklewright, L., Patrick, P., Purnell, S., Rowntree, C.J., & Smith, P. (2017). Pegylated-asparaginase during induction therapy for adult acute lymphoblastic leukaemia: toxicity data from the UKALL14 trial. *Leukemia*, 31(1), 58.

Patra, J.K., Das, G., Fraceto, L.F., Campos, E.V.R., Torres, M.P.R., Torres, L.S.A., Torres, L.A.D., Grillo, R., Swamy, M.K., Sharma, S., Habtemaria, M.S., & Shin, H.S. (2018). Nano based drug delivery systems: recent developments and future prospects. *Journal of Nanobiotechnology*, 16, 71. https://doi.org/10.1186/s12951-018-0392-8.

Poon, W., Kingston, K.R., Ouyang, B., Ngo, W., & Chan, W.C.W. (2020). A framework for designing delivery systems. *National Nanotechnology*, 15, 819–829. https://doi.org/10.1038/s41565-020-0759-5.

Prabhakar, P., & Banerjee, M. (2020). Nanotechnology in drug delivery system: Challenges and opportunities. *Journal of Pharmaceutical Sciences and Research*, 12(4), 492–498.

Sanna, V., & Sechi, M. (2020). Therapeutic potential of targeted nanoparticles and perspective on nanotherapies. *ACS Medicinal Chemistry Letters*, 11, 1069–1073. https://dx.doi.org/10.1021/acsmedchemlett.0c00075?ref=pdf.

Shi, C., Zhang, Z., Wang, F., & Luan, Y. (2018). Active-targeting docetaxel-loaded mixed micelles for enhancing antitumor efficacy. *Journal of Molecular Liquids*, 264, 172–178.

Sun, T., Zhang, Y.S., Pang, B., Hyun, D.C., Yang, M., & Xia, Y. (2014). Engineered nanoparticles for drug delivery in cancer therapy. *Angewandte Chemie International Edition*, 53, 12320–12364. http://doi: 10.1002/anie.201403036.

Yetisgin, AA., Cetinel, S., Zuvin, M., Kosar, A., & Kutlu, O. (2020). Therapeutic nanoparticles and their targeted delivery applications. *Molecules*, 25, 2193 http://doi:10.3390/molecules25092193.

Yin, H., Liao, L., & Fang, J. (2014). Enhanced permeability and retention (EPR) effect based tumor targeting: The concept, application and prospect. *JSM Clinical Oncology & Research*, 2(1), 1010.

4 Nanocarrier Used in Drug Delivery System

4.1 INTRODUCTION

Engineered nanoparticles (NPs) offer a lot of promise in terms of enhancing disease diagnosis and therapy specificity. Nanotechnology could assist in overcoming the restrictions of traditional delivery, from large-scale obstacles like biodistribution to smaller scale hurdles like intracellular trafficking, through cell-specific targeting, molecular transport to specific organelles, and other strategies. Low effectiveness, poor biodistribution, and a lack of selectivity characterize traditional pharmaceutical administration. Controlling medication distribution may be one way to get around these limitations and drawbacks. According to the current breakthroughs in nanotechnology, NPs (structures less than 100 nm in at least one dimension) have a lot of potential as drug carriers. Nanostructures offer unique physicochemical and biological properties that make them a useful material for biomedical applications (for example, enhanced reactive area and the ability to penetrate cell and tissue barriers). Nanocarriers with optimized physicochemical and biological properties are more easily absorbed by cells than larger molecules, making them potential delivery vehicles for bioactive substances that are already available. Liposomes, solid lipid nanoparticles (SLNs), dendrimers, polymers, silicon or carbon compounds, and magnetic NPs are some of the nanocarriers that have been studied as drug delivery systems (Figure 4.1). The process of conjugating the medication to the nanocarrier, as well as the strategy for targeting it, is crucial for a targeted therapy. A drug can be encapsulated in the nanocarrier or adsorbed or covalently bonded to its surface. Covalent linking has a benefit over other attachment methods in that it permits precise control of the number of drug molecules connected to the nanocarrier, i.e., the amount of therapeutic substance delivered.

For medical applications, biocompatible (able to integrate with a biological system without generating an immune response or creating any negative repercussions) and nontoxic nanocarriers are required (harmless to a given biological system). The negative effects of NPs are impacted significantly by their hydrodynamic size, shape, quantity, surface chemistry, administration method, immune system reaction (especially the route of uptake by macrophages and granulocytes), and bloodstream residency time. Because there are so many factors that might influence NP toxicity, calculating it can be difficult, which is why toxicological studies of any new DDS formulation are essential. In terms of particle size, however, some generalizations may be made: smaller particles have a bigger surface area, making them more reactive, and as a result, more dangerous. For in vivo applications, NPs with a hydrodynamic diameter of 10–100 nm are regarded to offer the optimum pharmacokinetic properties. Larger NPs are quickly opsonized and removed from the bloodstream

DOI: 10.1201/9781003252122-4

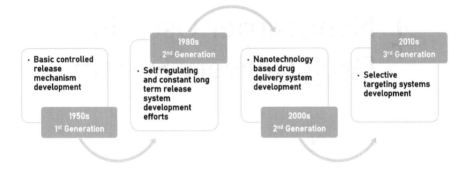

FIGURE 4.1   Progressive timeline history of drug delivery-based systems.

by reticuloendothelial system macrophages, but smaller NPs are subject to tissue extravasation and renal clearance (Figure 4.1).

4.2   CLASSES OF NANOPARTICLES

There are several subclasses of NPs, and some of the most prevalent ones are listed here (Mitchell et al., 2021). In terms of cargo, delivery, and patient response, each class offers a number of broad advantages and disadvantages (Figure 4.2).

A. **Lipid-based NPs:** The most typical lipid-based NPs are spherical platforms with at least one lipid bilayer enclosing at least one inner aqueous compartment. Formulation effortlessness, self-assembly, biocompatibility, high bioavailability, the ability to transport large payloads, and a variety of physicochemical properties that can be manipulated to modify their biological activities are all advantages of lipid-based NPs as a delivery vehicle. For these reasons, lipid-based NPs are the most common type of FDA-approved nanomedicine. Liposomes commonly feature surface alterations to extend their circulation and improve delivery because they can be quickly taken up by the reticuloendothelial system, which has enabled their clinical usage. Lipid nanoparticles (LNPs) – liposome-like structures frequently exploited for the transport of nucleic acids – are another notable subclass of lipid-based NPs. They are distinguished from standard liposomes by the formation of micellar structures within the particle core, a morphology that can be changed depending on formulation and synthesis conditions. Cationic or ionizable lipids that interact with negatively charged genetic material and promote endosomal escape, phospholipids for particle shape, cholesterol for stability and membrane fusion, and PEGylated lipids for improved stability and circulation are the four key components of LNPs. LNPs have become more relevant in personalized genetic therapy applications due to the efficacy of their nucleic acid delivery, as well as their ease of manufacturing, small size, and serum stability. Ionizable LNPs are an excellent platform for delivering these nucleic acid therapeutics because they have a near-neutral charge at physiological pH but become charged in acidic endosomal compartments, allowing for intracellular delivery. Despite these benefits, low drug loading and biodistribution, which results in significant absorption in the liver and spleen, can restrict LNP systems.

B. **Polymeric Nanoparticles (PNPs)** can be made from a number of sources, including natural and synthetic materials, monomers, and preformed polymers, allowing for a wide range of shapes and properties. Because they are biocompatible and have simple formulation parameters, they may be created to allow exact control of several NP characteristics. They are also good delivery vehicles. PNPs can also distribute drugs in a variety of ways. Therapeutics can be encapsulated in NP cores, entrapped in polymer matrixes, chemically linked to the polymer, or attached to the NP surface. PNPs are useful for co-delivery applications because they may convey a variety of payloads, including hydrophobic and hydrophilic substances, as well as cargos with diverse molecular weights, such as tiny molecules, biological macromolecules, proteins, and vaccines. PNPs can be made from a number of sources, including natural and synthetic materials, monomers, and preformed polymers, allowing for a wide range of shapes and properties. Because they are biocompatible and have simple formulation parameters, they may be created to allow exact control of several NP characteristics. They are also good delivery vehicles. PNPs can also distribute drugs in a variety of ways. Therapeutics can be encapsulated in NP cores, entrapped in polymer matrixes, chemically linked to the polymer, or attached to the NP surface. PNPs are useful for co-delivery applications because they may convey a variety of payloads, including hydrophobic and hydrophilic substances, as well as cargos with diverse molecular weights, such as tiny molecules, biological macromolecules, proteins, and vaccines. By modulating properties such as composition, stability, responsivity, and surface charge, the loading efficacies and release kinetics of these therapeutics can be precisely controlled. The most common forms of PNPs are nanocapsules (cavities surrounded by a polymeric membrane or shell) and nanospheres (solid matrix systems). Within these two large categories, NPs are divided further into shapes such as polymersomes, micelles, and dendrimers. Polymersomes are artificial vesicles, with membranes made using amphiphilic block copolymers. They are comparable to liposomes and are often locally responsive, but are reported to have improved stability and cargo-retention efficiency, making them effective vehicles for the delivery of therapeutics to the cytosol. Some polymers that are commonly copolymerized for these applications include poly(ethylene glycol) (PEG) and poly(dimethylsiloxane) (PDMS). Polymeric micelles, which are also typically responsive block copolymers, self-assemble to form nanospheres with a hydrophilic core and a hydrophobic coating: this serves to protect aqueous drug cargo and improve circulation times. Dendrimers are hyperbranched polymers with complex three-dimensional architectures for which the mass, size, shape, and surface chemistry can be highly controlled. Active functional groups present on the exterior of dendrimers enable conjugation of biomolecules or contrast agents to the surface, while drugs can be loaded in the interior. For these applications, charged polymers such as poly(ethylenimine)

(PEI) and poly(amidoamine) (PAMAM) are commonly used. Several dendrimer-based products are currently in clinical trials as theranostic agents, transfection agents, topical gels, and contrast agents. Charged polymers can be used to form non-dendrimer NPs as well. Polyelectrolytes are one such example: these polymers have a repeating electrolyte group, giving them charge that varies with pH. Polyelectrolytes have been incorporated in numerous NP formulations to improve properties such as bioavailability and mucosal transport. They are also inherently responsive and can be useful for intracellular delivery. Overall, PNPs are ideal candidates for drug delivery because they are biodegradable, water soluble, biocompatible, biomimetic, and stable during storage. Their surfaces can be easily modified for additional targeting – allowing them to deliver drugs, proteins, and genetic material to targeted tissues, which makes them useful in cancer medicine, gene therapy, and diagnostics. However, disadvantages of PNPs include an increased risk of particle aggregation and toxicity. Only a small number of polymeric nanomedicines are currently FDA approved and used in the clinic, but polymeric nanocarriers are currently undergoing testing in numerous clinical trials.

C. **Inorganic materials** such as gold, iron, and silica have been cast-off to produce nanostructured materials for various drug delivery and imaging applications. These inorganic NPs are precisely formulated and can be engineered to have a wide variety of sizes, structures, and geometries. Gold NPs (AuNPs), which are the most well studied ones, are used in various forms such as nanospheres, nanorods, nanostars, nanoshells, and nanocages. Additionally, inorganic NPs have unique physical, electrical, magnetic, and optical properties due to the properties of the base material itself. AuNPs are also easily functionalized, granting them additional properties and delivery capabilities. Iron oxide is another commonly researched material for inorganic NP synthesis, and iron oxide NPs make up the majority of FDA-approved inorganic nanomedicines. Magnetic iron oxide NPs – composed of magnetite (Fe_3O_4) or maghemite (Fe_2O_3) – possess superparamagnetic properties at certain sizes and have shown success as contrast agents, drug delivery vehicles, and thermal-based therapeutics. Other common inorganic NPs include calcium phosphate and mesoporous silica NPs, which have both been used successfully for gene and drug delivery. Quantum dots – typically made of semiconducting materials such as silicon – are unique NPs used primarily in in vitro imaging applications, but they show promise for in vivo diagnostics. Due to their magnetic, radioactive, or plasmonic properties, inorganic NPs are uniquely qualified for applications such as diagnostics, imaging, and photothermal therapies. Most have good biocompatibility and stability, and they fill niche applications that require properties unattainable by organic materials. However, little solubility and toxicity matters, particularly in heavy metal compositions, limiting their clinical applicability (Table 4.1; Figures 4.2 and 4.3).

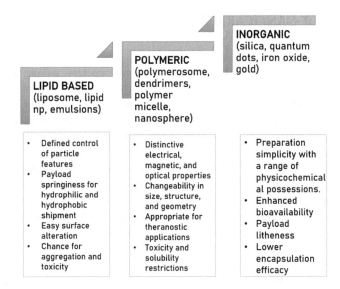

FIGURE 4.2 Characteristics overview of different classes of nanoparticles deployed in drug delivery.

TABLE 4.1
Momentous Evolution of Nanomedicine(Sur et al., 2019)

S. No	Year	Nanomedicine
1	1960	Liposomes
2	1976	Controlled release polymeric systems
3	1978	Dendrimers
4	1980	Targeted PEGylated liposomes
5	1994	Poly (lactic-co-glycolic acid) polyethylene glycol nanoparticle
6	1995	Doxil
7	1996	Ferumoxide
8	2005	Abraxane
9	2007	Genexol-PM
10	2008	CALAA-01 (targeted cyclodextrin- polymer hybrid)
11	2011	• SEL-068
		• BIND-014
12	2012	DXTL-TNP
	2014	BOX-BASP Nanoparticle
	2015 onwards	• Stimuli reactive nanoparticles
		• Mini machines
		• Site-specific directing nanoparticles
		• Biological intricacy

4.3 TYPES OF NANOCARRIERS

4.3.1 LIPOSOMES

Liposomes range in size from 30 nanometers to micrometers, having a phospholipid bilayer that is 4–5 nm thick. Liposomes have been studied extensively as carriers for small molecule medicines, proteins, nucleic acids, and imaging agents. To improve treatment efficacy and patient compliance, many delivery methods have been devised, including parenteral, pulmonary, oral, transdermal, ophthalmic, and nasal (Yadav et al., 2017).

The first description of swelling phospholipid systems was published in 1965 by a group of researchers. Within a few years, a variety of enclosed phospholipid bilayer structures made up of single bilayers were characterized, first as "bangosomes" and then as "liposomes." The concept that liposomes can entrap pharmaceuticals and be employed as drug delivery devices was established by early pioneers such as Gregoriadis and Perrie. The anticancer medication cytosine arabinoside was initially used to demonstrate the in vivo activity of liposome-entrapped medicines in animal models, with significant increases in the survival periods of mice carrying L1210 leukemia. It became a popular "model system" for evaluating the effects of a wide range of liposome properties on therapeutic results from then on.

Liposomes are designed to have the following optimal qualities (Yadav et al., 2017):

- Drug loading and drug release rate control.
- Overcoming liposomes' fast clearance.
- Drugs delivered intracellularly.
- Endocytosis of ligand-targeted liposomes through receptors.
- Release that has been triggered.
- DNA and nucleic acid delivery.

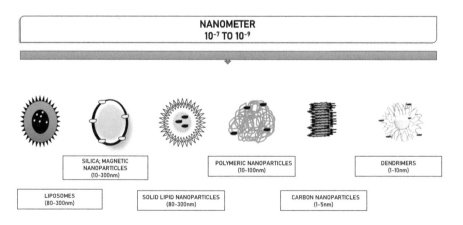

FIGURE 4.3 Different types of nanocarriers used in drug delivery.

Classification: Based on their size and number of bilayers, liposomes are classified as multilamellar vesicles (MLVs), large unilamellar vesicles (LUVs), and small unilamellar vesicles (SUVs). Based on their composition, they are classified as conventional liposomes (CLs), pH-sensitive liposomes, cationic liposomes, long circulating liposomes (LCLs), and immuno-liposomes. Based on the method of preparation, they are classified as reverse phase evaporation vesicles (REVs), French press vesicles (FPVs), and ether injection vesicles (EIVs). Based on their targeting ideas, they are classified as PEGylated liposomes, immunoliposomes, cationic liposomes, and thermosensitive liposomes.

Preparation Method: Thin-film hydration, ethanol injection, and double emulsion are some of the most prevalent manufacturing methods. Depending on the method of choice, the following steps are involved in preparation of MLVs or LUVs: size reduction, if necessary; preparation of the drug solution(s) and drug loading, which is combined with step 1 in the case of passive drug loading; buffer exchange and concentration, if necessary; sterile filtration or aseptic processing; lyophilization, if necessary; and packaging.

Stability: The stability of liposomes, which includes manufacture, storage, and administration, determines the therapeutic efficacy of the drug molecule. During the development and storage of an active molecule, a stable dosage form ensures the physical stability and chemical integrity of the active molecule.

Action Mechanism: Several processes are involved in the drug delivery function of liposomes:

- Liposomes adsorb to cell membranes, making contact with the membrane possible.
- Endocytosis: This process involves adherence of liposomes to the cell surface membrane, which is then engulfed and internalized into the liposomes.
- Fusion: Direct delivery of liposomal contents into the cytoplasm is achieved by fusing the lipid bilayers of liposomes with the lipoidal cell membrane via lateral diffusion and lipid intermingling.
- Lipid exchange: Lipid transfer proteins in the cell membrane easily recognize liposomes and cause lipid exchange because their lipid membranes are comparable to cell membrane phospholipids.

Applications: Site avoidance delivery, site-specific targeting, intracellular drug delivery, sustained release drug delivery, intraperitoneal administration, and immunological adjuvants in vaccines are only a few of the important therapeutic applications of liposomes in drug delivery.

- **Advantages:** Pharmacokinetics and pharmacodynamics are being improved and controlled.
- Toxicity has decreased.
- Drug action against intracellular infections is improved.
- Liposomes are utilized to select targets.
- Extracellular pathogens are more active than intracellular infections.

- **Disadvantages:** Lipid-based drug delivery systems are costly to manufacture, resulting in a high production cost.
- The price is high due to the high cost of the raw ingredients used in lipid excipients, as well as the expensive equipment required to boost production.
- Sterilization, short shelf life and stability, encapsulation efficacy, and removal from circulation via the reticuloendothelial system (RES) are all key challenges.

4.3.2 Nanoparticles Based on Solid Lipids

SLNs are matrix lipid particles made by substituting solid lipids for liquid lipids in an emulsion recipe. A few of the factors contributing to the growing interest in lipid-based systems include the fact that lipids improve oral bioavailability and minimize plasma profile variability, better characterization of lipoid excipients, as well as improved ability to solve the key concerns of knowledge transfer and manufacturing scale-up (Prabhakaran et al., 2011). These nanocarriers (50–1,000 nm) have piqued the interest of formulation scientists over the last two decades due to their compatibility and ability to penetrate various physiological barriers. Due to the poor mobility of drug molecules in a solid lipid matrix, solid lipids are gaining favor over liquid oils in the creation of controlled release nanoformulations. A solid lipid core is encased in a lipid monolayer to create these particles (Kammari et al., 2017). The use of biological lipids in the manufacturing of SLNs minimizes the risk of acute and chronic toxicity. SLNs with particle sizes of 120–200 nm can circumvent filtration in the liver and spleen.

Classification: The composition of lipid and oil mixtures determines the classification of nanostructured lipid carriers (NLCs) (Dhiman et al., 2021). There are three different sorts of NLCs:

i. Imperfect type: It is made by combining structurally diverse lipids that might cause crystal order to be distorted. Changing the saturation and amount of carbon atoms in lipids can enhance this distortion. As a result, the loading capacity increases.

ii. Amorphous: An amorphous matrix is created by combining lipids such as hydroxy octacosanyl hydroxystearate or isopropyl myristate with a solid lipid in amorphous type NLCs. The NLCs exist in an amorphous state as a result of these components, which avoids drug expulsion caused by modification during storage.

iii. Multiple oil-in-solid fat-in-water type: There are a variety of oil-in-solid fat-in-water types. The advantage of these NLCs is that they can hold more drugs and release them for a longer period of time.

Preparation Method: Different ways for making SLNs from lipid, emulsifier, and water/solvent are discussed below:

1. Homogenization under high pressure:
   - homogenization in a heat
   - homogenization in the cold

2. High-speed homogenization/ultrasonication:
   - Ultrasonication of the probe
   - Ultrasonic bathing
3. Evaporation of a solvent
4. Method of solvent emulsification-diffusion
5. The method of supercritical fluid
6. Method based on microemulsions
7. Using the spray drying process
8. Using two emulsions
9. The method of precipitation
10. Dispersion of film ultrasound

Stability: Changes in zeta potential, particle size, drug content, appearance, and viscosity as a function of time can be used to determine the physical properties of SLNs during long-term storage. Temperature and light appear to be the most important external conditions for long-term stability. For a dispersion to stay physically stable, the zeta potential should be higher than -60 mV in general. $20°C$ – Long-term storage did not result in drug-loaded SLN aggregation or loss of drug; $40°C$ – Most favorable storage temperature; $20°C$ – Long-term storage did not result in drug-loaded SLN aggregation or loss of drug; $50°C$ – A rapid increase in particle size was seen (Prabhakaran et al., 2011).

Action Mechanism: The following are the general drug release principles from LNPs:

- The partition coefficient of the drug has an inverse connection with drug release.
- Higher drug release is achieved by having a larger surface area due to smaller particle sizes in the nanometer range.
- When the drug is homogeneously disseminated in the lipid matrix, slow drug release can be achieved. It is dependent on the SLN type and drug entrapment model.
- The lipid's crystallinity and the drug's high mobility result in rapid drug release.

The degree of crystallization and the drug's mobility have an inverse connection. Large surface area, a high diffusion coefficient due to tiny molecular size, low viscosity in the matrix, and a short drug diffusion distance are all factors that contribute to a quick release. It was discovered that when particle size decreases, velocity increases.

Applications: Possible applications of SLNs are as follows: as an anticancer, for antimicrobial drug delivery, as gene carrier, in topical use, as a vaccine adjuvant, in antitubercular chemotherapy, and in bioimaging (Mishra et al., 2018).

Advantages: SLNs have a number of benefits over other nanocarriers (Mishra et al., 2018), including the ability to transport large amounts of information.

- Due to their nano size range, RES cells are unable to take up SLNs, allowing them to avoid spleen and liver filtration.

- Ensure that included medications have a high level of stability.
- Incorporation of both hydrophilic and lipophilic medicines is a possibility.
- Improve the bioavailability of compounds that are weakly water soluble.
- Sterilization and scaling up are simple processes.
- The immobilization of drug molecules within solid lipids protects sensitive pharmaceuticals from photochemical, oxidative, and chemical degradation, as well as reducing the risk of drug leakage.
- It is possible to dry using lyophilization.
- Make it possible for drugs to be released in a targeted and controlled manner.
- Compositional components that are biocompatible and biodegradable.

Disadvantages: Despite their many advantages, SLN-administered medications have a few drawbacks, including:

- SLNs are densely packed lipid matrix networks (perfect crystalline structure) with limited drug encapsulation space, resulting in low drug-loading capacity.
- During storage, the scattered phase begins to gel.
- A high water content (70–90%) can cause stability issues.
- The drug's loading in SLNs is determined by a number of parameters, including the drug's interaction with the lipid melt, the composition of the lipid matrix, drug's miscibility with the lipid matrix, and the drug's distribution or dissolution in the lipid matrix (Mishra et al., 2018).

4.3.3 POLYMERIC NANOPARTICLES

PNPs are small particles with a diameter of 1–1,000 nm that can be loaded with active chemicals or surface-adsorbed onto the polymeric core. The term "nanoparticle" is used to describe both nanocapsules and nanospheres, despite having different morphological structures. PNPs have showed considerable promise in the delivery of medications to specific locations for the treatment of a variety of ailments (Zielińska et al., 2020).

PNPs are particles or particulate materials with a one-dimensional size of at least 10–100 nm. One of the most commonly employed nanomaterials in nanomedicine is PNPs. The ability of PNPs to change current treatment is of great interest. Medication administration, including conjugation and entanglement of pharmaceuticals, prodrugs, stimuli responsive systems, imaging modalities, and theranostic, are all applications of PNPs. Biodegradable polymeric nanostructures (BPNs) have shown exceptional promise in a variety of therapeutic applications, including analysis, imaging, sedate delivery, cosmetic agents, organ embeds, and tissue design (Adhikari et al., 2021)

Classification: The following are the polymers based on their nature of origin (Sung and Kim, 2020):

i. Polymeric drug delivery methods have been developed using natural polymers such as arginine, chitosan, dextrin, polysaccharides, poly(glycolic acid), poly(lactic acid), and hyaluronic acid.

ii. Poly(2-hydroxyethyl methacrylate), poly(N-isopropyl acrylamide), poly(ethyleni-mine), and dendritic polymers are examples of **synthetic polymers**.

iii. alpha-hydroxy acids, polyanhydrides, poly(amides), poly(ester amides), poly(phosphoesters), poly(alkyl cyanoacrylates), poly(hyaluronic acids), and natural sugars like chitosan are all examples of **biodegradable and bioab-sorbable polymers**.

In comparison to biodegradable polymers made from natural polymers, synthetic bio-degradable polymers are preferred in drug delivery systems as they are immunogenic.

Preparation Method: Different methods for producing PNPs can be utilized depending on the type of medicine to be placed in them and their requirements for a specific administration route. The dispersion of premade polymers and the polymer-ization of monomers are the two basic techniques used in general. Techniques based on the polymerization of monomers can be used to load chemicals into PNPs with improved efficiency and in a single reaction step. The products are commonly obtained as aqueous colloidal suspensions, regardless of the mode of preparation used.

PNPs can be made in a variety of ways:

1. Nanospheres:
   • Evaporation of a solvent
   • Solvent diffusion/emulsification
   • Nanoprecipitation
   • Reverse salting-out/emulsification
2. Nanocapsules:
   • Nanoprecipitation

Stability: The adsorption of active molecules on the surface of NPs and the presence of adsorbed surfactants are two factors that can affect the stability of colloidal sus-pensions. Particle size, zeta potential, polymer molar mass distribution, drug content, and pH are some physicochemical parameters that may be used to assess the stability of polymeric colloidal suspensions. However, due to issues with low physicochemi-cal stability and long storage periods, commercial application of PNPs distributed in aqueous fluids may be limited. Particle aggregation, polymer chemical stability, drug or other raw materials employed during NP manufacturing, and early release of the active component are the key limits. It's also worth noting that liquid dose forms are susceptible to microbial contamination.

Action Mechanism: There are four main modes of drug delivery in controlled drug delivery systems: (i) rate-programmed drug delivery, in which drug diffusion from the system follows a specific release rate profile; (ii) activation-modulated drug delivery, in which drug release is induced by various factors such as physical, chemical, electrical, or biochemical modules; and (iii) feedback-regulated drug delivery, in which the rate of release is determined by biochemical substance. (iv) The rate of drug release is regulated by the specific targeting moiety, solubi-lizer, and drug moiety in site-targeted drug delivery systems, which is a complex process including numerous steps of diffusion rate and partitioning (Bennet and Kim., 2014).

Application: Medicinal applications include drug delivery – Treatment of vaginal diseases and in cancer treatment, bioimaging, biosensors, and stimuli reactive payload delivery.

Advantages: The advantages include tremendously small size, high volume-surface area ratio, adjustable pore, biodegradability, low or diminished cytotoxicity, long shelf life, high stability, and nontoxicity.

Disadvantages: Some polymers used in the delivery of therapeutic particles, including peptides, proteins, and nucleic acid medicines, are cytotoxic. Another significant problem is the time it takes for the polymer to respond and react, which is often slow. Barriers and constraints influencing the drug's efficiency include enzyme breakdown in the stomach, absorption across the intestinal epithelium, hepatic clearance, and accumulation in non-targeted organs. As a result, most polymeric drug delivery systems never make it to the clinic (Yadav et al., 2019).

4.3.4 DENDRIMER NANOCARRIERS

Dendrimers are novel polymeric nanoarchitectures characterized by hyper-branched 3D structure having multiple functional groups on the surface that increases their functionality and make them versatile and biocompatible. Their unique properties like nanoscale uniform size, high degree of branching, polyvalency, water solubility, available internal cavities, and convenient synthesis approaches make them promising agent for biological and drug delivery applications.

Because of their capacity to traverse cell membranes and lower the risk of early clearance from the body, dendrimers with homogeneous and well-defined size and shape are of particular interest in biomedical applications. They are an ideal carrier due to their great level of control on dendritic architecture. Recent improvements in synthetic chemistry and characterization techniques have allowed for the quick synthesis of a dendritic new carrier.

Classification: Dendrimers of various classes have been created using a range of core materials, branching units, and surface changes. Some of the dendrimers having different functionalities are PAMAM dendrimer, polypropylene imine (PPI) dendrimer, liquid crystalline (LC) dendrimers, core–shell (tecto) dendrimers, peptide dendrimers, glycodendrimers, hybrid dendrimers, and PAMAM-organosilicon (PAMAMOS) dendrimers.

Preparation Method: They are usually made by adding monomers over and again to a central polyfunctional core. There are several functional groups that make up the core. The most common methods for dendrimer synthesis are divergent and convergent methods (Wilczewska et al., 2012):

1. The activation of functional surface groups is the initial stage, followed by the addition of branching monomer units in the divergent method.
2. The convergent approach has two stages: a reiterative coupling of protected/deprotected branches to form a focal point functionalized dendron and a divergent core anchoring step to construct diverse multidendron dendrimers.

3. Other methods include the formation of "hypercores" and "branched monomers," "double exponential" growth, "lego" chemistry, and "click" chemistry.

Stability: The dendritic formulation helps to keep the chemicals inside the core stable by creating dynamic interior voids where neutral molecules and ions can be inserted to prevent deterioration.

Action Mechanism: Dendrimers can encapsulate pharmaceuticals within the dendritic structure or generate electrostatic/covalent interactions between drugs and terminal functional groups of dendrimers due to their precise 3D structure and many surface functional groups. There are two ways for drug distribution from drug–dendrimer conjugates. The first mechanism is based on the in vivo breakdown of covalent bonds between drug and dendrimer in the presence of enzymes or a bond-breaking environment. The second route of drug release involves changes in physical variables such as temperature and pH that are not influenced by external forces (Sherje et al., 2018).

Application: Dendrimers can be used for gene, protein, and enzyme delivery; they can also be used as nanoscale containers (nano-scaffolds), intracellular bioactive delivery, and microvascular extravasation.

Advantages:

- Increases the solubility of medicines that are very lipophilic.
- Chemical and physical qualities that can be altered.
- Multiple functional groups for targeted drug delivery.
- Covalently associating drugs.
- Acts like solubility enhancers.

Disadvantages:

- Not a good candidate carrier for hydrophilic drugs.
- Cellular toxicity.
- Elimination and metabolism are influenced by the generation and materials used.
- High cost of synthesis.

4.3.5 SILICA MATERIAL

Silica nanoparticles (SiNPs) are one of the most often employed nanoparticles in drug delivery applications because of its important properties such as large surface area, ease of functionalization, and biocompatibility. A porous variation, known as mesoporous silica nanoparticles (MSNs), adds features such as variable pore size and volume, resulting in a high drug-loading capacity. In the case of bacterial infections, SiNPs and their derivatives can be a useful tool for delivering antimicrobials to specific locations, potentially decreasing the impact of high medication dosage and its side effects.

Classification: SiNPs come in a variety of forms, including non-porous SiNPs, MSNs, hollow mesoporous silica nanoparticles (HMSNs), and core–shell silica, all of which can be modified on the surface. Because of its flexible and desired features, including high drug loading capacity, variable pore size and volume, ease of functionalization, and biocompatibility, MSN is a popular candidate for targeted drug delivery.

Preparation Method: A variety of methods can be used to make silica nanoparticles (SiNPs), which can range in size from 10 to 500 nm and have a variety of morphologies and physicochemical features. The following are the most regularly used SiNP synthesis methods (Selvarajan et al., 2020):

1. Stober's method.
2. The creation of oil-in-water (O/W) micelles or water-in-oil (W/O) reverse micelles which is a part of microemulsion method.
3. Method in the gaseous phase.
4. Method of precipitation.

Stability: Compared to niosomes, liposomes, and dendrimers, which do not require any external stabilization in the manufacture of MSNs, silica-based mesoporous nanoparticles are more resilient to external response such as deterioration and mechanical stress due to the strong Si–O link (Bharti et al., 2015).

Action Mechanism: MSNs allow a substantial number of (anticancer) medications to be loaded, allowing for passive targeting of the drugs in tumor tissues. PEGylation mechanisms allow therapeutic medicines to escape the RES, extending their circulation duration, availability, and biodistribution (Lombardo et al., 2019).

Application: Many medicinal applications, including cancer and antimicrobial therapies, have shown that SiNPs are a profitable alternative. Given the mounting threat of antimicrobial resistance, SiNPs' adaptability is particularly helpful for antimicrobial therapies, including biofilm treatment. In addition to the antibacterial action produced by the cargo, these NPs can target pathogens by a variety of mechanisms, including physical disruption to cell membranes, ROS generation, and endolysosomal load (Selvarajan et al., 2020).

Advantages:

- Well-defined surface properties.
- Size and shape tunability.
- High pore volume and surface area.
- High loading capacity and high bioavailability.

Disadvantages: The disadvantages include difficulty in well order preparation of particles and scattered size distribution.

4.3.6 Carbon Nanomaterials

As of their unique structural dimensions and physicochemical qualities, carbon-based nanoparticles (CBNs) have piqued attention in a variety of fields. These materials have showed greater drug-loading capacity, increased biocompatibility, and decreased immunogenicity thanks to their strong optical activity and large multifunctional surface area. The construction of biocompatible scaffolds and nano-medicines has been intensively investigated using functionalized CBNs. Specific moieties (e.g., functional groups, compounds, and polymers) of CBNs discovered to be useful for biomedical applications were chemically modified (Debnath and Srivastava, 2021).

Classification: Carbon atoms make up the majority of CBNs. They are categorized based on their geometrical structure and shape. Carbon nanotubes (CNTs), graphene, mesoporous carbon, nano diamonds, and fullerenes are the most often used carbon nanomaterials based on structure (Debnath and Srivastava., 2021). CNTs are divided into two classes based on the number of cylindrical graphene layers: single-walled carbon nanotubes (SWCNTs) and multi-walled carbon nanotubes (MWCNTs) (Chen et al., 2013).

Preparation Method: Three basic processes are routinely used to make CNTs:

1. Ablation with a laser
2. Chemical vapor deposition (CVD) with a thermal or plasma boost
3. Arc discharge (electric arc)

Micromechanical cleavage, epitaxial growth on SiC substrates, chemical reduction of exfoliated graphene oxide, CVD, liquid phase exfoliation of graphite, and unzipping of CNTs are some of the processes used to make graphene (Debnath and Srivastava., 2021). Depending on the intended use, each approach has demonstrated its strengths and limits.

Stability: Drugs are unable to pass through pores, yet they are finally dispersed throughout the carrier. Drugs, on the other hand, are not stable in this state because they do not bind or conjugate with carbon compounds and do not crystallize. CBNs are therefore immersed in a medication solution. The medications ultimately penetrate and disperse, bringing the situation to a state of equilibrium. Centrifugation was used to extract drug-laden CNMs from the solvent. In the solvent evaporation approach (Debnath and Srivastava, 2021), the solvent must evaporate after adsorption.

Application: CBNs in Gene Delivery and Peptide Delivery in Cancer Therapy: They have potential applications in the treatment of a variety of diseases, including cancer, genetic abnormalities, and the administration of bioactive in novel ways. Chemotherapeutics, antibiotics, proteins, DNA, RNA, vaccines, genes, and other drugs have all been successfully delivered using CNTs (both single- and multi-walled). Functionalized nano-GO, a graphene derivative, has been shown to be useful in delivering anticancer medicines without harming healthy cells (Mahor et al., 2021).

Advantages: The following are the exclusive properties of deploying CNMs (Mahor et al., 2021):

- Because of their supramolecular-stacking property, they can absorb a large amount of medication.
- CNMs can be used as theranostic materials because of their unique optical properties and ease of amalgamation with luminous substances.

- CNMs have a high heat conversion capability in the near-infrared range, making them ideal for photothermal therapy.
- Therapeutics can be released in a regulated manner using tunable surface chemistry.

Disadvantages:

- Toxicity
- Lack of safety
- tandardization of efficacy
- Formulation possibilities and other important issues that necessitate the creation of new clinical protocols and translation methodologies.

4.3.7 MAGNETIC NANOPARTICLES

Due to their improved biocompatibility and varied loading capabilities, magnetic nanoparticle-based drug delivery systems (MDDSs) are gaining prominence over other recognized systems.

Classification: MNPs can be classified as pure metals (such as cobalt, nickel, manganese, and iron), alloys, or oxides based on their magnetic characteristics. MDDSs are typically composed up of superparamagnetic iron-oxide NPs (Fe_3O_4, Fe_2O_3, etc.). Magnetic NPs are classified into four groups:

- Metals (Fe, Co, Ni)
- Oxides of metals (FeO, Fe_2O_3, Fe_3O_4)
- Alloys (FePt, FePd)
- Ferrites ($CoFe_2O_4$, $CuFe_2O_4$)

Preparation Method: Several alternative magnetic NP synthesis techniques have been published. Some are single-step procedures, while others are multi-step processes (McBain et al., 2008):

1. Wet precipitation
2. Co-precipitation – Reverse micelle mechanism
3. Chemical vapor condensation (CVC)
4. Thermal decomposition and reduction
5. Liquid phase reduction

Stability: Surface functionalization of magnetic NPs using chemical and biological methods improves their stability and biocompatibility. The regulated delivery of medications to target sites under external magnetic fields is the most intriguing element of magnetic NPs in drug delivery (Gul et al., 2019).

Action Mechanism: Magnetic NPs have been produced for cancer patients' localized medicine delivery. By acting as a drug carrier, these are guided to the tumor. Once the medicine has entered the patient's bloodstream, a magnetic field is used to keep the particles in the tumor's specific area.

Application: MNPs have a variety of applications, such as signal improvisation obtained from magnetic resonance imaging (MRI) techniques, endorsing the build-up of biotherapeutic amalgams, such as genes and peptides in gratifying microniches, and interceding the cancer cells and biofilms demolition by producing a local thermo-ablative effect, also known as magnetic hyperthermia (Williams., 2017).

Advantages: Magnetic (organic or inorganic) NPs have several advantages, including

- the ability to be visualized (superparamagnetic NPs are utilized in MRI);
- the ability to be directed and held in place by a magnetic field; and
- the ability to be heated in a magnetic field to induce medication release or produce tissue hyperthermia/ablation.

Disadvantages:

- As the application of an external magnetic field organizes the MNPs into a two-dimensional area, one of the constraints of magnetic NPs in drug administration is that they cannot be concentrated into a three-dimensional space.
- Once the magnetic field from outside is eliminated, it is difficult to keep the magnetic particles in the targeted organ.
- Another drawback is the time spent exposed to the magnetic field: because patients cannot be exposed to an external magnetic field indefinitely, treatment efficacy is limited by the frequency, strength, and duration of exposure to the magnetic field (Schneider and Ortega, 2021).

4.3.8 NANOBOTS

Nanobiotechnology adds a new level to robotics, resulting in the creation of nanorobots, also known as "nanobots." Nanobots will be miniaturized for entry into the body through the vascular system or at the end of catheters into various veins and other cavities in the human body, rather than executing treatments from outside the body. Nanobots are tiny robots that perform a single task and have a width of 50–100 nm. They can be used to deliver drugs very effectively. Drugs usually travel through the entire body before reaching the diseased location. The medicine might be targeted to a specific spot using nanotechnology, making it considerably more effective and reducing the risk of side effects.

The drug carriers have walls that are just 5–10 atoms thick and the inner drug-filled cell is usually 50–100 nm wide. When they detect signs of the disease, thin wires in their walls emit an electrical pulse which causes the walls to dissolve and the drug to be released (Mehta and Subramani, 2012).

Classification: A number of smart medical nanorobots have been developed and publicized to be effective in the management of tumor-targeting drugs for precise cancer therapy. (Huang et al., 2021):

1. Physical field-propelled nanomotors are categorized as follows:
   i. Light driven

      ii. Ultrasound driven
     iii. Magnetic field driven
  2. Chemical-propelled nanomotors
  3. Stimuli-responsive nanorobots:
       i. Endogenous stimuli-responsive nanorobots
      ii. DNA nanorobots triggered by aptamers
     iii. Exogenous stimuli-responsive nanorobots
     iv. Multi-stimuli-responsive nanorobots

Application: Applications range from detecting diseases by observing the production of specific enzymes around the infected area or in the blood, to drug delivery, which includes diseases such as diabetes and cancer, and reaching surgical targets of nanorobots in tumor elimination without causing harm to the surrounding area. Nanorobots also assist traditional methods of tumor diagnosis, therapy, or removal by providing complete data/maps of the area to be addressed, as well as monitoring human body behavior in normal conditions as a health check. Nanorobots have an unstoppable ability to simulate blood components and provide artificial blood, which aids in the treatment of a variety of ailments caused by a deficiency of one of the blood components. Examples of surgical nanorobots include nanocoated blades, suture nanoneedles, optical tweezers, nanorobots for cellular-level surgery, and nanorobots for destruction of cancerous tumors (Azar et al., 2020).

    Advantages: The amount and time of drug release can be easily controlled by controlling the electrical pulse. The walls dissolve easily and are therefore harmless to the body.

    Disadvantages: Nanorobots are still in their infancy in terms of research and development, and a major restriction is the potential for economic disruption as well as potential dangers to security, privacy, health, and the environment.

4.4   CONCLUSION

Initially, nanotechnology was primarily used to improve drug solubility, absorption, bioavailability, and controlled release, but it has since expanded to include a wide range of nano- dimensional tools that can be used to diagnose, precisely deliver at target, sense, or activate material in living systems. The efficacy of natural products has been considerably increased by using nanocarriers manufactured with gold, silver, cadmium sulfide, and titanium dioxide PNPs, as well as SLNs, nanogels, liposomes, micelles, iron oxide NPs, and dendrimers. The merging of therapy and diagnosis (theranostic) as an example of cancer as a disease model has been one of the key interests in the growth of nanomedicine in recent years. Since the 1990's, the number of FDA-approved nanotechnology-based products and clinical trials has increased dramatically, including synthetic polymer particles, liposome formulations, micellar NPs, nanocrystals, and many other nanotechnology-based products and clinical trials commonly accompanying drugs or biologics. Although future research will focus on regulatory frameworks for nanomedicines as well as safety/toxicity assessments, the method we identify and distribute medications in biological systems has already changed nanomedicine.

REFERENCES

Adhikari, C. (2021). Polymer nanoparticles-preparations, applications and future insights: a concise review. *Polymer-Plastics Technology and Materials*, 60(18), 1–29. https://doi.org/10.1080/25740881.2021.1939715.

Azar, A. T., Madian, A., Ibrahim, H., Taha, M. A., Mohamed, N. A., Fathy, Z., & AboAlNaga, B. M. (2020). Medical nanorobots: design, applications and future challenges. Control Systems Design of Bio-Robotics and Bio-Mechatronics with Advanced Applications, pp. 329–394. https://doi.org/10.1016/b978-0-12-817463-0.00011-3. ISBN 9780128174630.

Bennet, D., & Kim, S. (2014). Polymer nanoparticles for smart drug delivery. In: Sezer, A. D. (Ed.) Application of Nanotechnology in Drug Delivery, vol. 8. IntechOpen: New York, pp. 257–285. https://doi.org/10.5772/58422.

Bharti, C., Nagaich, U., Pal, A. K., & Gulati, N. (2015). Mesoporous silica nanoparticles in target drug delivery system: a review. *International Journal of Pharmaceutical Investigation*, 5(3), 124–133. https://doi.org/10.4103/2230-973X.160844.

Debnath, S.K.,, & Srivastava, R. (2021) Drug delivery with carbon-based nanomaterials as versatile nanocarriers. Progress and Prospects Frontiers in Nanotechnology, vol. 3. https://www.frontiersin.org/article/10.3389/fnano.2021.644564; https://DOI=10.3389/fnano.2021.644564.

Dhiman, N., Awasthi, R., Sharma, B. Bhupesh, Kharkwal, H., Kulkarni Giriraj, T. (2021) Lipid nanoparticles as carriers for bioactive delivery, *Frontiers in Chemistry*, 9. https://doi.org/10.3389/fchem.2021.580118.

Gul, S., Khan, S. B., Rehman, I. U., Khan, M. A., & Khan, M. I. (2019). A comprehensive review of magnetic nanomaterials modern day theranostics. *Frontiers in Materials*, 6. https://doi.org/10.3389/fmats.2019.00179. ISSN 2296-8016.

Huang, L., Chen, F., Lai, Y., Xu, Z., & Yu, H. (2021). Engineering nanorobots for tumor-targeting drug delivery: from dynamic control to stimuli-responsive strategy. *ChemBioChem*, 22, 3369–3380. https://doi.org/10.1002/cbic.202100347.

Kammari, R., Das, N. G., & Das, S. K. (2017). Nanoparticulate systems for therapeutic and diagnostic applications. Emerging Nanotechnologies for Diagnostics, Drug Delivery and Medical Devices, 2017, 105–144. https://doi.org/10.1016/B978-0-323-42978-8.00006-1.

Liu, P., Chen, G., & Zhang, J. (2022). A review of liposomes as a drug delivery system: current status of approved products, regulatory environments, and future perspectives. *Molecules*, 27, 1372. https://doi.org/10.3390/molecules27041372.

Lombardo, D., Kiselev, M. A., & Caccamo, M. T. (2019). Smart nanoparticles for drug delivery application: development of versatile nanocarrier platforms in biotechnology and nanomedicine. *Journal of Nanomaterials*, 2019, 1–26. https://doi.org/10.1155/2019/3702518.

Mahor, A., Singh, P.P., Bharadwaj, P., Sharma, N., Yadav, S., Rosenholm, J.M., & Bansal, K.K. (2021). Carbon-based nanomaterials for delivery of biologicals and therapeutics: a cutting-edge technology. *C*, 7, 19. https://doi.org/10.3390/c7010019.

McBain, S. C., Yiu, H. H., & Dobson, J. (2008). Magnetic nanoparticles for gene and drug delivery. *International Journal of Nanomedicine*, 3(2), 169–180. https://doi.org/10.2147/ijn.s1608.

Mehta, M., & Subramani, K. (2012). Nanodiagnostics in microbiology and dentistry. In: Subramani, K. & Ahmed, W. (Eds.), In Micro and Nano Technologies, Emerging Nanotechnologies in Dentistry, William Andrew Publishing, pp. 365–390. https://doi.org/10.1016/B978-1-4557-7862-1.00021-3.

Mishra, V., Bansal, K.K., Verma, A., Yadav, N., Thakur, S., Sudhakar, K., & Rosenholm, J.M. . (2018). Solid lipid nanoparticles: emerging colloidal nano drug delivery systems. *Pharmaceutics*, 10(4), 191. https://doi.org/10.3390/pharmaceutics10040191.

Mitchell, M.J., Billingsley, M.M., Haley, R.M. et al. (2021). Engineering precision nanoparticles for drug delivery. Nature Reviews Drug Discovery 20, 101–124. https://doi.org/10.1038/s41573-020-0090-8.

Nasir, S., Hussein, MZ., Zainal, Z., & Yusof, NA. (2018). Carbon-based nanomaterials/ allotropes: a glimpse of their synthesis, properties and some applications. *Materials*, 11(2):295. https://doi.org/10.3390/ma11020295.

Prabhakaran, E., Hasan, A., & Priyanka, K. (2011). Solid lipid nanoparticles: A review. 2.

Schneider-Futschik, E.K., & Reyes-Ortega, F. (2021). Advantages and disadvantages of using magnetic nanoparticles for the treatment of complicated ocular disorders. *Pharmaceutics*, 13(8), 1157. https://doi.org/10.3390/pharmaceutics13081157.

Selvarajan, V., Obuobi, S., & Ee, P. L. R. (2020). Silica nanoparticles—a versatile tool for the treatment of bacterial infections. *Frontiers in Chemistry*, 8. https://doi.org/10.3389/fchem.2020.00602.

Sherje, A.P., Jadhav, M., Dravyakar, B.R., & Kadam, D. (2018). Dendrimers: a versatile nano-carrier for drug delivery and targeting. *International Journal of Pharmaceutics*, 548(1), 707–720. https://doi.org/10.1016/j.ijpharm.2018.07.030.

Sung, Y.K., & Kim, S.W. (2020). Recent advances in polymeric drug delivery systems. *Biomaterials Research*, 24(1). https://doi.org/10.1186/s40824-020-00190-7.

Sur, S., Rathore, A., Dave, V., Reddy, K.R., Chouhan, R.S., & Sadhu, V. (2019). Recent developments in functionalized polymer nanoparticles for efficient drug delivery system. *Nano-Structures & Nano-Objects*, 20, 100397. https://doi.org/10.1016/j.nanoso.2019.100397.

Wilczewska, A. Z., Niemirowicz, K., Markiewicz, K. H., & Car, H. (2012). Nanoparticles as drug delivery systems. *Pharmacological Reports*, 64(5), 1020–1037. https://doi.org/10.1016/s1734-1140(12)70901-5.

Williams, H.M. (2017). The application of magnetic nanoparticles in the treatment and monitoring of cancer and infectious diseases. *Bioscience Horizons: The International Journal of Student Research*, 10, hzx009, https://doi.org/10.1093/biohorizons/hzx009.

Yadav, D., Sandeep, K., Pandey, D., & Dutta, R.K. (2017). Liposomes for drug delivery. *Journal of Biotechnology & Biomaterials*, 7(4). https://doi.org/10.4172/2155-952x.1000276.

Yadav, H.K.S., Almokdad, A.A., shaluf, S.I.M., & Debe, M.S. (2019). Polymer-based nanomaterials for drug-delivery carriers. *Nanocarriers for Drug Delivery*, 1, 531–556. https://doi.org/10.1016/b978-0-12-814033-8.00017-5. ISBN 9780128140338.

Yu-Cheng Chen, Xin-Chun Huang, Yun-Ling Luo, Yung-Chen Chang, You-Zung Hsieh, & Hsin-Yun Hsu (2013). Non-metallic nanomaterials in cancer theranostics: a review of silica- and carbon-based drug delivery systems, *Science and Technology of Advanced Materials*, 14, 4. https://doi.org/10.1088/1468-6996/14/4/044407.

Zielińska, A., Carreiró, F., Oliveira, A.M., Neves, A., Pires, B., Venkatesh, D.N., Durazzo, A., Lucarini, M., Eder, P., Silva, A.M., Santini, A., & Souto, E.B. (2020). Polymeric nanoparticles: production, characterization, toxicology and ecotoxicology. *Molecules (Basel, Switzerland)*, 25(16), 3731. https://doi.org/10.3390/molecules25163731.

5 Natural Product-Based Nanotechnology and Drug Delivery

5.1 INTRODUCTION

When compared to manufactured chemicals, most of the natural products have robust biological action, optimum adsorption, appropriate dispersal, acceptable breakdown, and abolition properties. Diverse natural goods stimulate a range of signal transduction trails to treat the diseases by modifying many targets, which has supplementary therapeutic probability than pharmaceuticals directed at a single location for multifactorial and complicated disorders. As a result, natural products not only have a good precursor structure but they also give immediate treatment.

Despite the fact that natural compounds have pharmacological action and therapeutic potential for human diseases, their application and development are hampered by their vulnerability to physiological media and low bioavailability. By enhancing bioavailability, targeting, and controlled release, nanotechnology provides an effective technique for efficient delivery of natural compounds to adapt to valuable clinical applications.

Biodegradability, biocompatibility, sustainability, renewable energy, and low toxicity are currently regarded as crucial elements in the manufacture and production of nanoformulations. In addition to the features listed above, biomaterials can, for the most part, be chemically modified, giving them unique and appealing properties for future nanomedicine applications. The antibacterial, antifungal, and cytotoxicity potential of nanoparticles, particularly silver nanoparticles, has been extensively researched in vitro (Figure 5.1).

Due to abundant presence of plants, plant-derived natural compounds have played a key role in medicine development. When it came to treating ailments, early humans recognized the therapeutic value of plants. These plants have been demonstrated to have medical efficacy in practice, as evidenced by the fact that they appear in a number of historical sources. Currently, around 60% of pharmaceutical provisions in the market are derivatives of botanical natural materials, and of those, approximately 80% of the world's inhabitants are contingent on traditional botanical preparations. The anticancer drug paclitaxel and its variants, the antimalarial drug artemisinin, and the cardio-cerebrovascular drug ginkgolide are among the "hot" drugs drawing international attention (Li et al. 2022).

- **Plant Secondary Metabolites: Classification and their Physicochemical Properties**

DOI: 10.1201/9781003252122-5

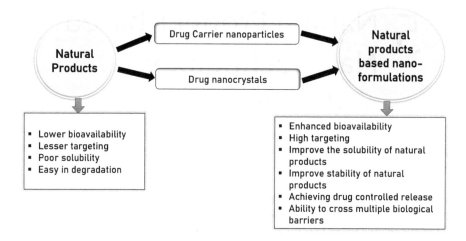

FIGURE 5.1 Intrinsic defects of natural products and reimbursements as nanoformulations.

Plants are a major source of a widespread variety of natural products with a varied series of chemical structures and health advantages. The primary metabolites and secondary metabolites are two types of plant-derived organic molecules. Primary metabolites (acyl lipids, phytosterols, proteins, nucleotides, organic acids, and sugars) are essential for plant survival because they play a critical role in photosynthesis; respiration; and normal growth, development, and reproduction. The adaptive therapeutic relevance of secondary metabolites was previously unknown; therefore, they were viewed as waste products. However, their medicinal value and vital activities in plants and human health are currently being assessed as a foundation of natural medicines, anticancer agents, antibiotics, insecticides, herbicides, allelopathic agents, UV protectants, pigments, scent, signaling molecules, and flavoring compounds.

Natural products, particularly secondary metabolites, have a wide structural and chemical variety, and because of their therapeutic potential, they continue to inspire new sightings in biology, chemistry, and medicine. These compounds have played a significant role in the creation of multi-targeted medications for the treatment of variety of human diseases, countering cancer, and they continue to do so.

- Plant phytochemical compounds are divided into primary and secondary metabolites reliant on their roles in elementary metabolic progressions.
- Because primary plant-based metabolites are engaged in basic life functions, they are found in all live cells in some form.
- Secondary plant metabolites, on the other hand, are products of subsidiary pathways such as the shikimic acid pathway.

The medical impact of herbals is targeted on secondary plant metabolites throughout research. Secondary plant metabolites have long been used in traditional medicine and folk medicine to treat a diversified ailment. They offered lead chemicals for the manufacture of drugs to treat a variety of disorders ranging from migraine to cancer in modern medicine. Secondary plant metabolites are categorized based on their chemical assemblies. They have been demonstrated to have a variety of biological effects, providing a scientific foundation for the use of herbs in traditional medicine in many ancient cultures. They have antibacterial, antifungal, and antiviral properties, and hence, can shield plants against contaminations. Besides, they contain crucial UV-absorbing chemicals, preventing major light damage to the leaves (Figure 5.2).

Phenolics, Alkaloids, Saponins, Terpenes, Lipids, and Carbohydrates are all examples of different classes of secondary plant metabolites (Table 5.1) (Hussein et al. 2018):

1. **Phenolics:** They are the most common type of secondary metabolite found in plants. They all have one or more phenol groups as a common feature, and they range in complexity from basic molecules with one aromatic ring to highly complex polymeric compounds. They are abundant in plants and play an important role in the color; taste; and flavor of many herbs, foods, and beverages. Pharmacologically, some phenolics are appreciated for their anti-inflammatory, anti-hepatotoxic, and phytoestrogenic effects, while others are insecticidal. Many phenolic compounds, particularly flavonoids, are powerful antioxidants and free radical scavengers.

2. **Alkaloids:** Alkaloids are known to possess diverse pharmacological effects that include analgesics, local anesthesia, cardiac stimulus, respiratory stimulus and easing, vasoconstriction, relaxation of muscles and toxicity, as well as anti-neoplastic, hypo- and hypertensive properties. The activity of alkaloids that have been reported in the literature is against herbivores, vertebrates' toxicity, cytotoxic action, the molecular targets, carcinogenic or mutagenic activity, antiviral and allelopathic, antibacterial as well as antifungal properties.

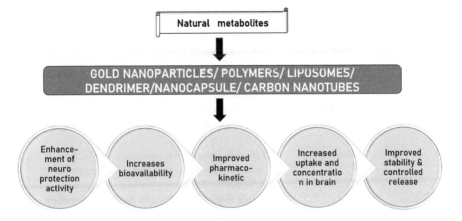

FIGURE 5.2 Nanoformulations used to improve the effectiveness of natural compounds.

TABLE 5.1

Characteristics of Different Classes of Secondary Metabolites

Secondary Metabolites	Sub Classes	Characteristics
Phenolics	Simple phenolics	Antibacterial, antiviral, antifungal, anti-inflammatory, anticancer, anti-anaphylactic, anti-mutagenic, choleretic, and bronchodilators effects have been observed in vitro
	Tannins and xanthones	Tannin-containing medications are antidiarrheal and have been used as antidotes for heavy metal and alkaloids poisoning
	Coumarins	The most notable biological activity documented for coumarins includes anti-inflammatory, anticoagulant, anticancer, and anti-Alzheimer's
	Flavonoids	The group is renowned for its anti-inflammatory and anti-allergic capabilities, as well as antithrombotic and vasoprotective properties, tumor inhibition, and gastric mucosa protection
	Chromones	Associated with antioxidant, antimicrobial, anticancer, and anti-inflammatory activities
	Stilbenes	Chemopreventive, anti-obesity, antidiabetic, and neuroprotective properties
	Lignans	Some show antimicrobial and antifungal activities, while others showed cytotoxic activities
Alkaloids	Nicotine	Has tranquilizing properties
	Caffeine	It acts as a diuretic and stimulates the respiratory, cardiovascular, and neurological systems
	Vinblastine	It has been used to treat diabetes and high blood pressure
Saponins		They have been reported to show antitumor, piscicidal, molluscicidal, spermicidal, sedative, expectorant, and analgesic properties and they also act as antitussive agent
Terpenes	Hemiterpenes	Anticarcinogenic, antimalarial, antiulcer
	Monoterpenes	As analgesics, anti-itching agents, and antihelmintics
	Sesquiterpenes	Diuretic, analgesic, and anti-inflammatory
	Diterpenes	Diaphoretics, antirheumatics, and anti-feedant properties
	Sester-terpenes	Anti-inflammatory, cytotoxic, anticancer, antimicrobial, and anti-biofilm actions
	Triterpenes	Anti-inflammatory, antirheumatic activities and insecticide
Lipids	Fixed oils	Potent antioxidants and anti-inflammatory
	Waxes	Anti-inflammatory, anti-aging, and wound healing actions
	Essential oils	Antiseptic, antimicrobial, analgesic, sedative, anti-inflammatory, spasmolytic, and locally anesthetic remedies
Carbohydrates		To treat inflammatory digestive disorders, particularly where ulceration is present

3. **Saponins:** These soap-like chemicals have the capacity to reduce surface tension. They promote hemolysis of blood erythrocytes in vitro and generate foam in water solutions.

4. **Terpenes:** They are among the biggest and most diverse group of plant secondary compounds. Terpenes' medicinal properties are supported by numerous in vitro, animal, and clinical trials and show anti-inflammatory, antioxidant, analgesic, anticonvulsive, antidepressant, anxiolytic, anticancer, antitumor, neuroprotective, anti-mutagenic, anti-allergic, antibiotic, and antidiabetic attributes.

5. **Lipids:** Fixed oils, waxes, essential oils, sterols, fat-soluble vitamins (such as vitamins A, D, E, and K), phospholipids, and other naturally occurring compounds make up lipids. Despite the fact that lipids are considered fundamental plant metabolites, new research has proven that they have medicinal properties.

6. **Carbohydrates:** Although carbohydrates are primary metabolites, glycosylation connections allow them to be integrated into several secondary metabolites. Carbohydrates play a significant biological and structural role in plants, and some members, such as mucilage, have therapeutic properties. Mucilage, a viscous sticky substance generated by practically all plants and some microbes, protects plant membranes by thickening them. When mucilage comes into direct contact with mucous membrane surfaces or skin, it serves as a local demulcent or emollient.

The requirement for new drugs?

- There is an increase in cases of drug resistance, for example, antibiotics and cancer chemotherapies.
- Traditional medicine is growing in underdeveloped nations, despite pharmaceutical companies moving away from drug development based on natural product research.
- In the field of biotherapeutics, there are some exciting new advances.

Delivery of natural products?

- Natural products' bioavailability, biodistribution, therapeutic efficacy, and stability can all be improved by using drug delivery systems.
- Multiple components are introduced into drug delivery systems to provide a variety of responsibilities (such as imaging) as well as therapy.

Why delivery of biotherapeutics?

- Provides a variety of administration options.
- Molecule targeting has been improved.

Challenges in producing nanoformulations based on natural products

While there have been many nanomedicine-related research and tests, only a small number have progressed to market-related review and even fewer have received final approval. According to some accounts, the transfer of foundational science into clinical practice was less than 10%. As a result, medications that transit through the "valley of death" do not appear to be practical. This results in a time-consuming, protracted, and pointless series of evaluations, raising the overall cost of healthcare. The explanations for this unfavorable situation could be found in a variety of domains and procedural aspects (Hamid and Manzoor, 2020).

- One of the major issues is the behavior of nanoparticles in vivo, which is expected to differ from their behavior in vitro. Cellular interactions, tissue transfer, diffusion, and biocompatibility are the main issues that need to be thoroughly investigated utilizing various animal (in vivo) models. Such tests are neither straightforward nor inexpensive to conduct in order to offer appropriate confirmation of effectiveness and protection.
- The heterogeneity and diverse character of tumors is another stumbling block for tumor-targeted nanoformulations in particular. Different gene expression profiles, molecular patterns, and degrees of drug resistance between malignancies may obstruct tumor-targeted NP penetration and efficacy (Martin et al. 2020). This difficulty could result in a failed clinical trial (despite encouraging preclinical findings in animals) and rejection of the nanoformulations under investigation.
- Other parameters that necessitate exact expert experimentation include drug penetration into tumors, efficacy of drug release into target cells, and the quality of drug-loaded nanoparticles (Dancy et al. 2020).
- This comprehensive research may not be possible in all biomedical laboratories. Another source of anxiety is due to time and money restrictions.
- Another roadblock to nanoformulation acceptance could be the multifunctional structure and operation of some nanoformulations. Many investigational nanoformulations feature a hybrid structure with diagnostic and therapeutic components that are independent. Different trials are needed to show that such systems are protected, and the long-term biocompatibility of such systems is unknown. Regulatory agencies have varying constraints on this topic, and long-term safety of these theranostic nanoformulations will require time-consuming and expensive regulatory research. Many traditional approaches to nanoformulation synthesis are now insufficient and require further development and optimization.
- The potential toxicity of nanoparticle delivery systems for natural chemicals is a major concern. This is a serious worry with nanoparticles, partially because they can traverse biological membranes such as cellular membranes, and in some situations, the blood–brain barrier (BBB) (Enrico, 2019)
- Another issue that can stymie the development of sufficient stocks of nanoformulations for market approval is batch-to-batch variation. Updating production processes and very precise characterization of nanoformulations are likely to be time-consuming, costly, and difficult.
  - Nanoformulations of natural metabolites (Table 5.2).
  - Naturally obtained compounds conjugated with nanocarriers for the treatment of various diseases.

TABLE 5.2
Various Nanoformulations of Natural Metabolites (Kashayap et al. 2021)

Class	Nanocarrier	Description
Lipid-based systems	Liposomes	Liposomes are lipid bilayer vesicles with a membranous lipid bilayer mostly made up of natural and/or manufactured phospholipids that enclose an aqueous phase. The solvents that are freely floating inside the liposomes are encapsulated by the liposomes
	Solid lipid nanoparticles	The nanospheres have a solid lipid core with an average core diameter of 50–1,000 nm
	Double emulsions	It is a bi-phasic system (aqueous and oil) in which one phase is dispersed as minute droplets with diameters ranging from 0.1 to 100 m in the other phase
Protein-based systems	Gelatin	Collagen hydrolysis is used to make it. It is commonly utilized for cancer treatment delivery due to its great biocompatibility. To improve drug release from nanoparticles by lowering drug insolubility at elevated temperatures, gelatin-based nanostructures must be cross-linked with cross-linkers such as genipin or glutaraldehyde
	Milk proteins	It has important qualities like the ability to interact with macro- and micro-molecules, a suitable surface for self-assembly, and great gelation capabilities, all of which help to improve medication bioavailability
	Zein proteins	Prolamin protein, which contains hydrophobic amino acids, proline, and glutamine, is abundant in zein. Films and coatings contain a lot of zein. A variety of medications have been encapsulated using zein nanoparticles
	Albumin-based nanoparticles	Albumin is an ideal material for drug delivery systems because of its great stability over a wide pH range and higher temperatures, as well as preferential uptake by tumor and inflamed tissue, biodegradability, low toxicity, and immunogenicity
	Polypeptide nanoparticles	Elastin-like polypeptides (ELPs), which consist of alternating hydrophobic blocks and cross-linking domains, are the most widely manufactured polypeptide nanoparticles. ELPs have a distinct phase behavior that promotes recombinant expression, protein purification, and nanostructure self-assembly
	Sericin	Sericin is composed of 35% sheet and 63% random coil, with no helical component, resulting in the protein's unfolded state. Antioxidant and anticancer properties are found in sericin nanoparticles. The fibroblasts are unaffected by sericin nanoparticles

(Continued)

TABLE 5.2 (*Continued*)

Various Nanoformulations of Natural Metabolites (Kashayap et al. 2021)

Class	Nanocarrier	Description
Carbohydrate-based systems	Cyclodextrins	Due to the presence of glucopyranose, cyclodextrins have a truncated cone form. Cyclodextrins are important for building an efficient medication delivery system because of their unique features
	Chitosan	Chitosan is also more biocompatible and responsive to changes such as ionic cross-linking and covalent binding, allowing it to be used to create a variety of nanomaterials such as nanoparticles, films, nanogels, and fibers. Chitosan has features that make it a good candidate for use in theranostic nanomedicine
	Other polysaccharides	Derivable reactive groups found on polysaccharides can be used to functionalize nanomaterials, making tiny medicines and diagnostic agents easier to conjugate
	Multi-biopolymers systems	Nanoparticles" ability to connect to various organic molecules has resulted in their important roles as medication and vaccine carriers into target cells or tissues

Compounds that are physiologically active are frequently found to be highly water soluble but have low absorption (such as flavonoids, tannins, and terpenoids), and in some cases, have a high molecular weight (such as polysaccharides). When evaluated in vivo, they are unable to readily traverse lipid membranes, resulting in poor absorption and loss of biological activity. Furthermore, when exposed to normal cells, some chemicals are extremely hazardous. Delivery methods can be used to improve absorption, minimize toxicity, and boost selectivity of some of these chemicals in this regard (Table 5.3).

- Application of natural product-based nanodrugs (Li et al. 2021):
  1. Used to treat cancer.
  2. Used to treat diabetes mellitus.
  3. Alzheimer's disease, Parkinson's disease, and Huntington's disease are examples of neurodegenerative disorders that can be treated.
  4. Used in the treatment of cardiovascular diseases.

TABLE 5.3

Certain Natural Compounds Being Inspected with Delivery Systems (Obeid et al. 2017)

S. No.	Plant/Constituents Delivery System	Biological Activity	Delivery System Used	Efficacy of the Delivery System
1.	Curcumin	Anticancer	Liposomes	The systemic residence period is long, and the entrapment efficiency is great
2.	Curcumin	Anticancer and antioxidant	Phytosomes	Improved antioxidant activity and bioavailability
3.	Curcumin	Anticancer	Emulsion system	To help with absorption
4.	Curcumin	Anticancer and antioxidant	Transferosomes	Enhanced permeation
5.	Curcumin	Anti-inflammatory	Micropelletization	To allow for long-term release and selective locus targeting
6.	Quercetin	Anticongestion and antianxiety	Liposomes	Efficacy, bioavailability, and adverse effects all had been improved
7.	Quercetin	Anti-inflammatory and antioxidant	Microspheres	Improved permeation
8.	Quercetin	Antioxidant	Emulsion system	To enhance permeation
9.	Ginkgo biloba	Brain activator	Nanoparticles	Improve the flow of blood and metabolism in the brain
10.	Ginkgo biloba	Antiasthmatic, antidiabetic, and cardioprotective	Phytosomes	To boost efficacy
11.	Wogonin	Anticancer	Liposomes	To extend the duration of the activity
12.	Embelin	Antifertility and antibacterial	Phytosomes	To improve solubility

5.2 CONCLUSION

Besieged distribution of naturally occurring compounds and phytochemicals by deploying nanoparticles or nanocarriers can improve their bioavailability and biodistribution significantly. Natural compounds and phytochemicals are usually low in toxicity; the only issue is that large doses of these natural substances cause adverse effects, which lead to limited patient compliance. Natural products and phytochemicals offer a range of benefits, including relative pharmacological safety and pharmacological efficacy against a variety of illnesses and malignancies via many targets' molecular pathways.

REFERENCES

Dancy, J. G., Wadajkar, A. S., Connolly, N. P., Galisteo, R., Ames, H. M., Peng, S., & Kim, A. J. (2020). Decreased nonspecific adhesivity, receptor-targeted therapeutic nanoparticles for primary and metastatic breast cancer. *Science Advances*. https://doi.org/10.1126/sciadv.aax3931.

Enrico, C. (2019). Nanotechnology-based drug delivery of natural compounds and phytochemicals for the treatment of cancer and other diseases. *Studies in Natural Products Chemistry*, 91–123. https://doi:10.1016/b978-0-444-64185-4.00003-4.

Hamid, Rabia, Manzoor, Ifrah. (2020). Nanomedicines: Nano Based Drug Delivery Systems Challenges And Opportunities. https://doi.org/10.5772/intechopen.94353.

Hussein, R.A., & El-Anssary, A.A. (2018). Plants secondary metabolites: the key drivers of the pharmacological actions of medicinal plants. In: Herbal Medicine. IntechOpen. https://doi.org/10.5772/intechopen.76139.

Kashyap, D., Tuli, H. S., Yerer, M. B., Sharma, A., Sak, K., Srivastava, S., Pandey, A., Garg, V.K., Sethi, G., & Bishayee, A. (2019). Natural product-based nanoformulations for cancer therapy: opportunities and challenges. Seminars in Cancer Biology. https://doi:10.1016/j.semcancer.2019.08.014.

Li, Zhe, Zhao, Tingting, Li, Jiaxin, Yu, Qingying, Feng, Yu, Xie, Yicheng, & Sun, Peng. (2022). Nanomedicine based on natural products: improving clinical application potential. *Journal of Nanomaterials*. 2022. https://doi.org/10.1155/2022/3066613.

Martin, J.D., Cabral, H., Stylianopoulos, T., & Jain, R.K. (2020). Improving cancer immunotherapy using nanomedicines: progress, opportunities and challenges. *Nature Reviews Clinical Oncology*, 1–16. https://doi.org/10.1038/s41571-019-0308-z.

Obeid, M.A., Al Qaraghuli, M.M., Alsaadi, M., Alzahrani, A.R., Niwasabutra, K., & Ferro, V. A. (2017). Delivering natural products and biotherapeutics to improve drug efficacy. *Therapeutic Delivery*, 8(11), 947–956. https://doi.org/10.4155/tde-2017-0060.

6 Nanoparticles in Diagnosis, Detection, and Imaging

6.1 INTRODUCTION

Nanomedicine is the use of nanotechnology in medicine and healthcare, and it has been utilized to treat some of the most common ailments, such as cardiovascular disease and cancer. At the nanoscale, nanomaterials contain unique optical, electrical, and/or magnetic properties that can be employed in a variety of applications, including electronics and medical. Nanomaterials are one-of-a-kind in that they have a high surface area to volume ratio. Nanomaterials, unlike other large-scaled manufactured objects and systems, are regulated by quantum mechanics rather than conventional physics and chemistry. One of the most important steps in the healthcare process is disease diagnosis. To avoid "false negative" cases, all diagnosis should be prompt, accurate, and specific. In vivo imaging is a non-invasive technique that identifies signs or symptoms within a patient's live tissues, without the need to undergo surgery. A previous improvement in diagnostic imaging techniques is the use of biological markers that can detect changes in the tissues at the cellular level. The aim of using a biological marker is to detect illnesses or symptoms, thereby serving as an early detection tool. In addition to diagnosis, imaging is vital not only for detecting potential toxic reactions but also for controlled drug release research, evaluating drug distribution within the body and closely monitoring the progress of a therapy. Potential drug toxicity can be reduced with the possibility of monitoring the distribution of drugs around the body and by releasing the drug as required. Anatomic and functional imaging, as well as effective medication delivery, are all possible using NPs that have been conjugated to diverse biomolecules. NPs are delivered in three steps: (i) systemic localization while avoiding reticuloendothelial system (RES) sequestration, (ii) extravasation from intratumoral capillaries, and (iii) diffusion and penetration into malignant cells.

Currently utilized medical imaging contrast agents are mostly tiny compounds with a fast metabolism and a non-specific distribution, which might lead to unwanted hazardous side effects. Because nanoparticles (NPs) have lower toxicity and greater permeability and retention effects in tissues, this is where nanotechnologies offer the most significant contribution in the field of medicine, by generating more strong contrast agents for practically all imaging modalities. The scale Molecular imaging includes optical bioluminescence, optical fluorescence (FL), targeted ultrasound, molecular magnetic resonance imaging (MRI) and spectroscopy (MRS), single-photon emission computed tomography (SPECT), and positron emission tomography

(PET). The inherent strengths and limits of each modality have prompted the active development of multimodal systems for synergistic imaging, such as SPECT/CT, PET/CT, optical/CT, and PET/MRI.

- **Nanoparticles in Fluorescence Imaging**

  Because of its adaptability, selectivity, sensitivity, rich contrast, and high-resolution capabilities, bioimaging utilizing nanomaterials has contracted a lot of attention in biomedical research with the discovery of new functional materials. Optical imaging could previously only be resolved to a restricted range (200 nm). However, with the improvement of fluorescent imaging methods such as photo-activated localization microscopy (PALM) and stimulated emission depletion (STED) microscopy, the resolution increased dramatically. Bioimaging with nanomaterials primarily employs three techniques: (i) fluorescent nanomaterials are injected into cells and tissues to make them fluorescent; (ii) targeted bioimaging; and (iii) nanomaterials are used as sensors to sense cellular biochemical species that are not fluorescent intrinsically (Ghosh and Sharma, 2020).

  Fluorescence is a type of luminescence in which a substance absorbs radiations before emitting light of a certain wavelength. Fluorophores are molecules that have the ability to emit light when they absorb light. Fluorescence imaging is a non-invasive method for visualizing many biological processes in living systems. It encompasses a wide range of findings, including protein expression, gene expression, and cell–tissue interactions.

  - This technique entails visualizing fluorescent proteins and dyes in order to comprehend numerous molecular events that occur in living cells, and hence, it serves as a possible tool for biochemical applications. Fluorescence microscopy involves labeling materials with a fluorescent probe and then shining a strong light on them.
  - At a specific wavelength, the tagged fluorophore absorbs and then emits.
  - As a result, a high-contrast image can be obtained on a black backdrop.

    Fluorescence imaging is the most widely used tool to study biological processes. There are two types of fluorescence imaging namely intrinsic and extrinsic fluorescence imaging.

    - The first kind of imaging usually refers to the fluorescence emission by intrinsic fluorophoric species such as tryptophan residues in proteins and NADH in tissues.
    - The second type of imaging is based on extrinsic fluorescence, which is exhibited by synthetic dyes and probes, nanomaterials, sensors, and so on. They basically help in the detection of species, which are not visible through direct fluorescence imaging (Table 6.1).

- **Nanoparticles in MRI**

  Metals (gold, silver, and cobalt) and metal oxides (Fe_3O_4, TiO_2, and SiO_2) are among the materials used in nanoparticles with potential MRI medical uses (Blasiak et al., 2013).

  - **Iron-Based Nanoparticles:** The so-called small and ultrasmall superparamagnetic iron oxide (USPIO) and superparamagnetic

TABLE 6.1

Different Types of Nanomaterials Frequently Used in Bioimaging and Their Features (Ghosh and Sharma, 2020)

S. No.	Nanomaterials	Characteristics	Reported Examples
1.	Fluorescent metallic nanoparticles	Better photostability, improved low detection limits, targeted detection, high quantum yield, and clinical applicability are among the advantages. Because of the interaction between the surface plasmon of metal nanoparticles and the dipole moment of fluorophores, metallic nanoparticles enhance the fluorescence characteristics of fluorophores in their vicinity	Gold nanoparticles (AuNPs), silver islands/scaffolds, nanoclusters made from silver, gold, and copper
2	Magnetic nanoparticles	Have biocompatibility, superparamagnetic characteristics, and the ability to customize surface functionalization	Aminopropyl silica coated γ-Fe_2O_3
3	Quantum dots	When compared to typical organic and inorganic fluorophores, QDs have higher photostability, brightness, and tunable light emission. Functionalization improves water solubility and allows for more precise targeting	CdS QDs, ZnO QDs doped with Gd, bioconjugated CdSe/ZnS QDs, silica-coated Fe_3O_4/CdTe quantum dots, polymer-coated QDs
4	Hydrogels or hydrophilic polymers	Their biodegradability, 3D cross-linking network, biocompatibility, sensitivity, nontoxicity, and fast gel to sol transformation in response to biological stimuli are all advantages	Supramolecular metallo-hydrogel based on ruthenium (II) tris(bipyridine) complex, Poly(ethylene glycol)-co-poly (ethylene oxide); also called pluronic hydrogel
5	Polymer dots	Rapid fluorescence decay rates, high quantum yield, large absorption cross-sectional area ($104\,cm^2$), and low chromophore density; extraordinary emission rates equip the particle to operate as efficient imaging probes due to small particle size, strong cellular uptake through endocytosis, nontoxicity, and photostability They feature a brilliant fluorescence that often extends into the near-infrared range	Conjugated polymers

(Continued)

TABLE 6.1 (*Continued*)

Different Types of Nanomaterials Frequently Used in Bioimaging and Their Features (Ghosh and Sharma, 2020)

S. No.	Nanomaterials	Characteristics	Reported Examples
6	Silicon-based nanomaterials	High surface area to volume ratio, unique chemical, biodegradable, electrical, and optical properties, noncytotoxic, high photostability, brightness, biocompatibility, and biodegradability	Silicon nanowires (SiNWs) incorporated with glutaric acid, SiNPs capped with allylamine, SiNWs coated with AuNPs, silica having gadolinium oxide (Gd2O3) NPs, silica doped with dye-encapsulated in gadolinium silylated shell
7	Carbon dots	Noncytotoxic, have appropriate photostability and chemical inertness, and are easy to modify on the surface	Highly luminescent C-dots fabricated from citric acid, C-dot surface passivated with polyethyleneimine, C-dot SiO_2 nanoparticles further functionalized with PEG molecules, carbogenic nanodots doped with iron oxide
8	Various other carbon-based nanomaterials	At different excitation wavelengths, distinct colored fluorescence emission is produced, and the photoluminescence is size-dependent	Carbon containing nanomaterials such as graphene oxide, graphene QDs, nanodiamonds, graphite oxide, and carbon nanotubes
9	Micelles, dendrimers, and lipid nanoparticles	Micelles have a highly loadable surface and homogeneous size, as well as improved fluorescence brightness, retention time, biocompatibility, nontoxicity, and improved accumulation	Indocyanine green and polycaprolactone (ICG-PCL) micelle, supramolecular micelles that involve perylene-diimide and poly(D, L-lactide)-b-poly(ethyl ethylene phosphate)
		Dendrimers' small size makes them easily endocytosed, and they are highly fluorescent with a high molar absorbance, which means they have better photostability, brightness, localization, and resolution for bioimaging	Dendritic nanoprobes conjugated with cyanine dye, polyamide amine (PAMAM)
		Lipid NPs are frequently employed in bioimaging because of their bioavailability, low toxicity, and large-scale synthesis	Lipid NPs are labeled with various probes and dyes (emitting in NIR region)

iron oxide (SPIO) are the most common and first to be used in MRI nanoparticles. Magnetite (Fe_3O_4) and maghemite (Fe_2O_4) are the most common monocrystalline components of SPIONs. Because iron oxide has a low saturation magnetization, it necessitates the usage of big particles in order to achieve adequate MRI contrast.

- **Core–Shell Nanoparticles:** In imaging applications, there are two types of core/shell nanoparticles: inorganic/organic and inorganic/inorganic. Silica (SiO_2) is the most common organic shell, whereas inorganic materials include a variety of metals. Many inorganic core–shell nanoparticles, such as Au@Ag, Au@Co, Au@Pt, Au@TiO_2, Au@Fe_2O_3, Ni@Ag, Fe@Ag, Ni@Pt, Co@Au, Fe@Pt, LaF3@Eu or -$NaYF_4$:Yb^{3+}, and Er^{3+}/-$NaYF_4$:Yb^{3+}, have been constructed.

- **Other Nanoparticles:** Other than iron oxide-based nanoparticles, cobalt (Co), gold (Au@Fe), and platinum (Pt@Fe) have potential clinical use in MRI and/or CT. Because they have a much higher saturation magnetization value than iron, they have a much larger effect on proton relaxation for copolymer, core diameter, and 28 nm particle diameter, providing better MR contrast and allowing smaller particle cores to be used without compromising MR sensitivity than iron oxide in the same concentration. Cobalt is probably the most commonly utilized metal.

- **Nanoparticles in Computed Tomography Imaging**

  The significance of computed tomography (CT) as one of the most widely used radiological methods in biomedical imaging has accelerated the development of nanoparticles as next-generation CT contrast agents. Because of their many benefits over conventional contrast agents, such as prolonged blood circulation time, controlled biological clearance pathways, and specialized molecular targeting capabilities, nanoparticles are predicted to play a large role in the future of medical diagnostics. In terms of availability, efficiency, and cost, CT is one of the most convenient imaging/diagnostic tools utilized in hospitals today. CT is not usually thought of as a molecular imaging modality, in contrast to other imaging modalities such as PET, SPECT, and MRI. Much recent research has focused on the production of nanoparticles for use as CT contrast agents in blood pools and for specialized molecular imaging applications.

  CT is currently one of the most widely used radiological technologies in the field of biomedical imaging. Because of the intrinsic contrast between electron-dense bones and the more permeable surrounding soft tissues, CT allows for better visibility of bone structures. CT, on the other hand, has trouble discriminating between soft tissues with identical densities. CT contrast agents were developed to increase vascular contrast and delineate soft tissue structures with similar or equivalent contrast characteristics.

  Antibodies, peptides, and other ligands can be conjugated to the surface of nanoparticles to create active targeting agents that can selectively aggregate on certain cells or tissues. By boosting the local accumulation of nanoparticles in regions of interest, molecularly targeted particles have the potential to greatly increase CT contrast and specificity. The use of molecularly targeted CT contrast agents broadens CT's role beyond its current structural imaging capabilities, allowing it to perform functional and molecular imaging as well. To avoid quick clearance by the kidneys or uptake in the liver, the ideal nanoparticle should be larger than 15 nm and less than 200 nm to avoid filtration in the spleen (Shilo et al., 2012) (Table 6.2).

TABLE 6.2
Different Classes of Nanomaterials to be Used as Contrasting Agents

S. No.	Nanomaterials	Characteristics
1.	Iodine-based CT contrast agents	Iodine molecules with a high atomic number ($Z = 53$) are effective in absorbing X-rays; nevertheless, the small size of iodine molecules allows for very quick imaging times due to rapid kidney clearance. To solve this restriction, larger sized iodine-based contrast agents with longer blood circulation times were created. Liposomes, polymers, and micelles are used to make these "soft" nanoparticles
2.	Liposome-based CT contrast agents	Given the relative instability of liposomes in biological environments, creating a liposome contrast agent necessitates extra caution. Blood half-life time in hours has been observed for liposomes larger than 100 nm
3.	Polymeric CT contrast agents	Physical entrapment or covalent linkage of core molecules to polymeric chains is used to make polymeric CT contrast agents. Blood half-life period has been recorded in minutes for polymers with sizes ranging from 30 to 400 nm. They must be properly engineered so that they do not decompose and clump together after being injected into the bloodstream
4.	Metal nanoparticles as CT contrast agents	CT contrast agents made of metal nanoparticles Metal nanoparticles offer a variety of physical, chemical, and biological features that make them ideal candidates for CT contrast agents. As previously stated, the higher the contrast agent's atomic number, the better the CT contrast (proportional to Z3). Tantalum, gold, and bismuth (atomic numbers 73, 79, and 83, respectively) are newly suggested metals with substantially greater atomic numbers than the currently utilized iodine. As a result, the proposed metals may cause more X-ray attenuation. Furthermore, because the size of the metal nanoparticles can be carefully regulated, the CT signal, which is directly proportional to the number of contrast molecules in a voxel, may be optimized. Gold nanoparticles (GNPs) have received a lot of attention among metal nanoparticles.

- **Nanoparticles in PET/SPECT Imaging**

  PET and SPECT imaging methods can be extremely useful in the creation of new nanoparticle drug delivery systems, and these studies also provide the chance to design extraordinary new diagnostic and therapeutic radiopharmaceuticals. The dynamic synergy of PET and nanotechnology combines PET's sensitivity and quantitative nature with nanomaterials' multifunctionality and tunability, which can assist solve some of the field's fundamental obstacles. SPECT and PET are non-invasive nuclear imaging modalities that offer tremendous opportunities in early lesion detection, patient screening and stratification, and individualized treatment monitoring and dose optimization due to their high detection sensitivity, quantifiability, and limitless depth of penetration, as well as advances in radiotracer development (Goel et al., 2017). For example, radiolabeled iron oxide nanoparticles (IONPs) signal for both MRI and PET at the same time, possibly overcoming the limits of each modality.

  PET radionuclide labeled nanoparticles includes (Xing et al., 2014)

  - **Carbon-Based Nanoparticles:** Carbon nanotubes (CNTs), graphene oxide nanoparticles, fullerenes, and perfluorocarbon nanoemulsions are among the most widely used carbon-based nanoparticles in biological applications. CNTs are hollow nanostructures with lengths ranging from a few hundred nanometers to several micrometers that are well-ordered. Single-walled carbon nanotubes (SWCNTs) with diameters ranging from 0.4 to 2 nm and multi-walled carbon nanotubes (MWCNTs) with diameters ranging from 2 to 100 nm are examples of CNTs. For PET imaging, positron emitting radionuclides can be conjugated or even incorporated into CNTs.

  - **Liposomes:** Liposomes are an effective substrate for the selective delivery of imaging moieties because of their unique qualities of encapsulating hydrophobic agents in the lipid shell, hydrophilic agents in the aqueous core, and amphiphilic compounds scattered within the hydrophobic/hydrophilic domains. In vivo PET imaging, Emmetiere and co-workers found that ^{18}F radiolabeled liposomes had fast clearance, low non-specific binding, high signal-to-background activity ratios, and little toxicity to the kidneys and bone marrow.

  - **Gold Nanoparticles:** Due to their appealing features, such as size controllability, high biocompatibility, and ease of surface modification, gold nanoparticles (GNPs) are tempting for the development of imaging agents. GNPs have showed considerable promise in PET, CT, Raman spectroscopy, and photoacoustic imaging (PAI) up to this point.

  - **Metal Oxide Nanoparticles** have been widely used in the development of PET imaging probes. Another important class of nanoparticle for PET imaging is radiolabeled iron oxide. Standard superparamagnetic iron oxide (SSPIO) with a diameter of 60–150 nm, ultra–small superparamagnetic iron oxide (USPIO) with a diameter of 5–40 nm, and mono crystalline iron oxide (MION) with a diameter of 10–30 nm are the three types of IONPs. The SPIONPs stand out among these IONPs because of their biocompatibility and inherent capacity to promote surface modification, making them appealing as multifunctional imaging agents.

- **Micelles:** Polymer micelles have recently gained popularity for PET imaging due to their great stability and biocompatibility. The conjugation of water-soluble copolymers with lipids (such as polyethylene glycol–phosphatidyl ethanolamine, PEG–PE) can produce a specific type of polymeric micelle.
- **Dendrimers:** Dendrimers come in a variety of sizes, molecular weights, and chemical makeups. Dendrimers are useful scaffolds or vehicles for the creation of imaging probes because of their high loading capacity and flexibility in manipulating the polymer structure. Because the DOTA chelator in dendrimers can easily be labeled with positron emission nuclides like ^{64}Cu, the newly discovered dendrimers could provide a possible PET platform.

• **Nanoparticles in Ultrasound Imaging**

  Because of its inherent advantages over other imaging technologies, ultrasonography (US) is commonly used in clinical imaging. Because of their unique capabilities and great performance, NP-based imaging and therapeutic modalities have been widely exploited. Organic NPs, inorganic NPs, and hybrid NPs are the three types of NPs that can be classified based on their structural configuration. For US imaging or therapy, organic and inorganic NPs have distinct advantages and disadvantages. Organic NPs are biocompatible, biodegradable, and have a high acoustic responsibility. Their stability, on the other hand, is low for long-term US imaging or therapy. Inorganic NPs are known for their great stability and biocompatibility, yet their breakdown rates are modest. Inorganic NPs also have the specific physiochemical characteristics that cause US irradiation (Li et al., 2020) (Figure 6.1 and Table 6.3).

• **Nanoparticles in Multimodality Imaging**

  Modern molecular imaging techniques can be classified into five major categories: (i) optical bioluminescence and fluorescence imaging techniques, (ii) PET and SPECT, (iii) CT, (iv) MRI, and (v) optical or ultrasound imaging (OI or US). In recent years, there has been tremendous interest in developing techniques combining molecular imaging with MRI, CT, PET, SPECT, optical imaging, or PAI to evaluate anatomical and physiological processes in vivo, so-called multimodality or multimodal molecular imaging.

  The role of nanotechnology in molecular imaging is fourfold. Nanoparticles can act as signal amplifiers, resulting in higher contrast indices and enhanced sensitivity. The large surface area can be

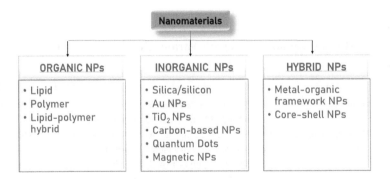

FIGURE 6.1 Classification of nanoparticle for ultrasound-based imaging.

TABLE 6.3
Nanoparticles for Different Ultrasound Imaging

Single Modality		Multiple Modality	
NP Types and Modification	**Function**	**NP Types and Modification**	**Function**
PFP/PLGA-PEG-FA NPs	Targeted US imaging by phase shift	The nanodroplets loaded with 10-hydroxycamptothecin and Fe$_3$O$_4$	Exhibiting MR/PA/ US imaging and drug releasing after irradiation of low intensity focused US
Mesoporous CaCO$_3$ NPs	US imaging as well as imaging-guided SDT	SPIO NPs surface-modified with the antibody herceptin	Exhibiting targeted US/PA imaging and simultaneous PTT of breast cancer
Exosome-like silica NPs	Exhibiting significant US-impedance mismatch	PLGA nanosystem loading ZnPc and PFH	Exhibiting dual-modal PA and US imaging
NPs with liquid PFOB as the core and PLGA-COOH, PLGA-PEG-COOH as the shell	Offering good tumor-selective US enhancement	Hyaluronic acid NPs modified with indocyanine green and encapsulated with MnO$_2$	Exhibiting imaging and improving PDT efficacy

Abbreviations: FA, ferulic acid; MSNs, mesoporous silica nanoparticles; PEG, poly(ethylene glycol); PFP, perfluoropentane; PLGA, poly(lactic-co-glycolic acid); PTT, photothermal therapy; US, ultrasonography.

functionalized with different targeting moieties, creating a multifunctional nanoplatform for targeted detection of different diseases. A big advantage of using nanoprobes over the traditional biological moieties is the competence for multimodality (Table 6.4).

TABLE 6.4

Characteristics of Nanoparticles with Various Building Blocks for Multimodal Imaging (Liu et al., 2019)

S. No.	Types	Characteristics	Imaging Modality
1.	Dendrimers	High drug loading, highly branching, monodispersed, and synthetic macromolecules	CT/MRI/NIR
2.	Polymeric micelles	The hydrophilic coating around the core, the appropriate size with a narrow distribution, the biocompatible polymer shell, the reduced toxicity, the good modulation, and the thermodynamic stability are all advantages	CT/MRI
3.	Liposomes	Self-assembly, simplicity of preparation, biodegradability, reduced toxicity and adverse effects, and ease of loading of hydrophilic and hydrophobic payloads	CT/MRI
4.	Iron NPs	Magnetic and catalytic characteristics, MRI contrast agent, size and shape control, and biocompatibility	MRI
5.	Gold NPs	Controllable size and form; simple surface modification; higher absorption and biocompatibility	CT/PAT/ SERS
6.	Carbon-based NPs	Structural stiffness, high drug loading, and a unique electrical property	Raman/PAT

6.2 CONCLUSION

X-ray, ultrasound, CT, nuclear medicine, and MRI are all well-known imaging modalities that are commonly employed in biochemical and medical research. However, these approaches can only look at alterations on the tissue surface later in disease progression, while they can be enhanced by using nanotechnology-based contrast and targeting agents to improve resolution and specificity by showing the diseased spot at the tissue level. Because nanoparticles have lower toxicity and greater permeability and retention effects in tissues, this is where nanotechnologies offer the most significant contribution in the field of medicine, by generating more strong contrast agents for practically all imaging modalities. The size of nanoparticles has a big impact on their biodistribution, blood circulation half-life, and cellular effects.

REFERENCES

Blasiak, B., Van Veggel, F.C.J.M., & Tomanek, B. (2013). Applications of nanoparticles for MRI cancer diagnosis and therapy. *Journal of Nanomaterials*, 2013, 1–12. https://doi.org/10.1155/2013/148578.

Emmetiere, F., Irwin, C., Viola-Villegas, N.T., Longo, V., Cheal, S.M., Zanzonico, P., Pillarsetty, N., Weber, W.A., Lewis, J.S., & Reiner, T. (2013). (18)F-labeled-bio orthogonal liposomes for in vivo targeting. *Bioconjugate Chemistry*, 24(11), 1784–1789. https://doi.org/10.1021/bc400322h.

Goel, S., England, C.G., Chen, F., & Cai, W. (2017). Positron emission tomography and nano-technology: a dynamic duo for cancer theranostics. *Advanced Drug Delivery Reviews*, 113, 157–176. https://doi.org/10.1016/j.addr.2016.08.001.

Li, L., Guan, Y., Xiong, H., Deng, T., Ji, Q., Xu, Z., Kang, Y., & Pang, J. (2020). Fundamentals and applications of nanoparticles for ultrasound-based imaging and therapy. *Nano Select*, 1(3), 263–284. https://doi.org/10.1002/nano.202000035.

Liu, M., Anderson, R., Lan, X., Conti, P.S., & Chen, K. (2019). Recent advances in the development of nanoparticles for multimodality imaging and therapy of cancer. *Medicinal Research Reviews*, 40(3), 909–930. https://doi:10.1002/med.21642.

Paluszkiewicz, P., Martuszewski, A., Zaręba, N., Wala, K., Banasik, M., & Kepinska, M. (2022). The application of nanoparticles in diagnosis and treatment of kidney diseases. *International Journal of Molecular Sciences*, 23, 131. https://doi.org/10.3390/ijms23010131.

Pratiwi, F.W., Kuo, C.W., Chen, B.-C., & Chen, P. (2019). Recent advances in the use of fluorescent nanoparticles for bioimaging. *Nanomedicine*. https://doi.org/10.2217/nnm-2019-0105.

Shilo, M., Reuveni, T., Motiei, M., & Popovtzer, R. (2012). Nanoparticles as computed tomography contrast agents: current status and future perspectives. *Nanomedicine*, 7(2), 257–269. https://doi.org/10.2217/nnm.11.190.

Sim, S., & Wong, N. (2021). Nanotechnology and its use in imaging and drug delivery (Review). *Biomedical Reports*, 14(5). https://doi.org/10.3892/br.2021.1418.

Sundar Ghosh, K., & Sharma, A. (2020). *Fluorescent Nanomaterials for Cellular Imaging*. https://doi.org/10.5772/intechopen.93278.

Xing, Y., Zhao, J., Shi, X., Conti, P.S., & Chen, K. (2014). Recent development of radiolabeled nanoparticles for PET imaging. *Austin Journal of Nanomedicine & Nanotechnology*, 2(2), 1016.

Yadollahpour, A., Mansoury Asl, H., & Rashidi, S. (2017). Applications of nanoparticles in magnetic resonance imaging: a comprehensive review. *Asian Journal of Pharmaceutics*, 11, S7–S13.

7 Nanoparticle Application in Non-Parenteral Applications

7.1 INTRODUCTION

The medication's route of administration is determined by the drug's pharmacokinetics and pharmacodynamic profile, as well as convenience and compliance. As a result, understanding the features of various routes and strategies associated with them is critical. The route of drug administration is simply defined as the method via which a medicine is injected into the body for the purposes of diagnosing, preventing, curing, or treating various diseases and disorders. A drug must get into contact with the tissues of organs and cells of tissues in some way for it to have the desired therapeutic effect, and in order for this to happen, the drug must be delivered properly.

The route of administration of a medication has a direct impact on drug bioavailability, which dictates the pharmacological effect's onset and durability. Many factors can influence the route of administration that you choose, including

- patient's comfort state;
- desired onset of action;
- patient's cooperation;
- the drug's nature, as some medications are only effective through one route, such as insulin;
- the patient's age; and
- the effect of gastric pH, digestive enzymes, and first-pass metabolism.

7.2 CLASSIFICATION OF VARIOUS ROUTES OF DRUG ADMINISTRATION

Local and systemic are the two types of administration routes. The local route is the most straightforward method of delivering a medicine to the exact location where it is needed. When systemic absorption of a drug is sought, drugs are often supplied through one of two routes: enteral or parenteral.

The medicine is absorbed through the gastrointestinal tract via the enteral route, which includes oral, sublingual, and rectal administration. Injection routes (e.g., intravenous, intramuscular, and subcutaneous), inhalational, and transdermal routes, on the other hand, do not entail drug absorption via the gastrointestinal tract (par = around, enteral = gastrointestinal) (Raj et al., 2019) (Figure 7.1).

DOI: 10.1201/9781003252122-7

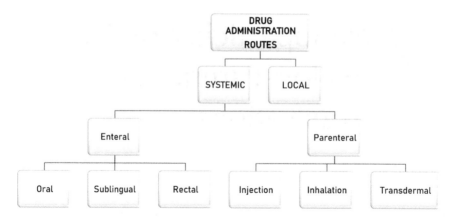

FIGURE 7.1   Different routes of drug delivery.

The main routes of drug administration include the following:

  i. **Oral Route:** This is the most common method of medication administration. It is the first choice for drug delivery when practicable, as it is both convenient and cost-effective. Orally given drugs are swallowed after being inserted in the mouth. Most orally administered medications are rapidly absorbed into the bloodstream from the gastrointestinal tract, within the limits of the drug's physicochemical qualities. Antacids for heartburn and ezetimibe for cholesterol absorption decrease are examples of medications that are taken orally for their local effects within the gut. Oral agents must be able to resist the stomach's acidic environment and penetrate the intestinal lining before reaching the bloodstream. Tablets, capsules, suspensions, and solutions are the most common oral dose forms.
 ii **Topical Route:** Drugs are applied topically to the skin or mucous membranes of the eye, ear, nose, mouth, vaginal canal, and other areas for local effect. This method allows for a high local concentration of the medicine while avoiding any effects on the broad circulation. Drugs that are absorbed into the bloodstream after local delivery, on the other hand, may have systemic effects. Creams, ointments, liniments, and drops are commonly used for topical treatments.
iii. **Transdermal route:** Because the medication is housed in a patch that is absorbed via the skin, the transdermal method is usually referred to as "the patch." Drugs that are delivered this way must have a high lipophilicity. This method of absorption is sluggish, yet it is conducive to providing long-lasting effects. Some transdermal patches use special slow-release matrices to keep medication concentrations consistent, similar to those of a continual intravenous (IV) infusion. Transdermal patches help reduce gastrointestinal absorption issues that are typical in people who take oral drugs. Fentanyl patches for severe pain management, nitroglycerin transdermal patches for preventing episodes of angina in persons with coronary artery disease, nicotine patches for smoking cessation, and other drugs are administered by this manner.

iv **Inhalational Route/Pulmonary Route:** Inhalation is a frequent method of drug delivery for both local and systemic effects. Using both powder aerosols (e.g., salmeterol xinafoate) and pressurized metered-dose aerosols carrying the medicine in liquid inert propellant, this delivery mechanism is particularly useful for the direct treatment of asthmatic disorders (e.g., salbutamol sulfate inhaler). Drugs can be inhaled as gases (e.g., nitrous oxide) and then diffused over the alveolar membrane into the bloodstream. This is how volatile anesthetics like ether, halothene, and methoxyflurane are administered. When a medicine is administered as a gaseous, aerosol mist, or ultra-fine solid particle, the lungs provide a good surface for absorption. As a result, action takes place quickly. Another benefit is that plasma concentration may be changed quickly.

v. **Injection Routes:** This is the second most popular method of medication delivery. They mostly entail injecting the medicine as a solution or suspension into the body using a syringe and needle at various places and depths. As a result, there is a risk of infection, discomfort, and local irritation during administration. Injection routes of medication administration are commonly used in the following situations:

- rapid effect is urgently needed as in emergency situations;
- the patient is too ill or unconscious for oral route to be employed;
- the drug is orally ineffective as it is being destroyed or not absorbed from the gut;
- an injection is the only way for the drug to reach its require site of action;
- there is a need to maintain a steady blood level of a drug.

  The surrounding tissue or site must be as clean as possible, and all tools used must be clean and sterile, according to the most significant factors or standards in all injection routes. Subcutaneous (SC), intramuscular (IM), and intravenous (IV) injections are the most prevalent. Intra-arterial (IA), intrathecal (IT), intraperitoneal (IP), intravitreal, and other routes are utilized less frequently (Tables 7.1 and 7.2).

TABLE 7.1
Various Routes of Drug Administration Via Injection

Injection Routes	Characteristics
Subcutaneous (SC)	Hypodermic is a term used to describe the administration of medication through the skin. The terms subdermal and hypodermal are interchangeable
Intramuscular (IM)	Administration within a muscle
Intradermal (ID)	Administration within the dermis
Intravenous (IV)	Administration within or into a vein or veins
Intra-arterial (IA)	Administration within an artery or arteries
Intrathecal (IT)	Administration within the cerebrospinal fluid at any level of the cerebrospinal axis, including injection into the cerebral ventricles
Intraperitoneal (IP)	Administration within the peritoneal cavity
Intravitreal	Administration within the vitreous body of the eye

TABLE 7.2
Nanoparticles for Targeting Different Sites (Yildirimer et al., 2011)

S. No.	Target	Nanocarriers	Characteristics Features
1.	*Lung targets:* Because of the non-invasive nature of inhalation therapy, the lung's enormous surface area, drug localization/accumulation within the pulmonary tissue, and avoidance of first-pass metabolism, the lung is an ideal target for drug delivery	Polymeric nanoparticles	Polymeric NPs are biocompatible, surface changeable, and have the ability to release drugs over an extended period of time. They show promise in the treatment of pulmonary diseases such asthma, chronic obstructive pulmonary disease (COPD), tuberculosis (TB), and lung cancer, as well as extrapulmonary diseases like diabetes
		Carbon nanotubes (CNTs)	SWCNTs and MWCNTs are two types of carbon nanotubes, with the former being more cytotoxic as SWCNTs have a higher surface area than the multi-layered option
		Silica (SiO_2) nanoparticles	In comparison to their crystalline pendants, which are classified as class 1 carcinogens, silica NPs are regarded "safe" in modest doses (20 g/mL). However, silica NPs showed agglomerative potential in vitro at a dose of 25 g/mL and dose-dependent cytotoxicity on A549 cells at a critical concentration of 50 g/mL
		Silver nanoparticles	Occupational inhalation of airborne particles during manufacturing is the most prevalent route of lung exposure to silver NPs (AgNPs). Inhaled NPs can also move from their original deposition site (e.g., the lungs) to other tissues

(Continued)

TABLE 7.2 (Continued)
Nanoparticles for Targeting Different Sites (Yildirimer et al., 2011)

S. No.	Target	Nanocarriers	Characteristics Features
2.	*Dermal targets:* Topically administered NPs have the ability to permeate the skin and enter the systemic circulation, causing systemic effects. It is subjected to a variety of non-specific environmental assaults in the air, as well as specific and possibly hazardous compounds included in creams, sprays, and garments	Silver nanoparticles	Ag intake and topical treatment can produce argyria, a benign disorder characterized by a gray–blue coloring of the skin and liver caused by Ag particle deposition in the basal laminae of these tissues
		Titanium dioxide (TiO₂) nanoparticles	Cell type—dependent TiO$_2$ toxicity was discovered in vitro, influencing cellular activities such as cell proliferation, differentiation, mobility, and apoptosis
		Silica nanoparticles	A size-related increase in cytotoxicity was discovered in cell-based toxicity studies Smaller particles (100 nm) had a higher cellular absorption efficiency, which is associated with enhanced cytotoxicity
		Gold nanoparticles	The amount of AuNP taken up by cells is a function of time, particle size, and concentration. Smaller NPs went deeper into the tissue than larger ones, which are gathered mostly in the epidermis and dermis at the surface
3.	*Liver targets:* The liver is particularly prone to NP toxicity because it is the location of first-pass metabolism, and it has been found to store given drugs even after exposure has ended. The significance of a thorough assessment of NP-mediated hepatocellular toxicity remains paramount	Gold nanoparticles	The toxicity of AuNP is affected not only by the features stated above, such as surface functionalization, but also by the route of administration Particles administered intraperitoneally had a considerably higher rate of adverse consequences than those delivered intravenously, according to research
		Silver nanoparticles	Particle concentration, size, shape, and the ability to deplete cells of antioxidants are all factors that influence the degree of toxicity
		Silica nanoparticles	Silica NPs' hepatotoxic potential, resulting in mononuclear inflammatory cell infiltrates at the portal area and hepatocyte destruction. Linked to the promotion of pro-inflammatory cytokine production after unsuccessful phagocytosis of bigger silica NPs (>100 nm)
		Quantum dots	Smaller particles (20 nm) extravasating through capillary fenestrae large enough in the liver (100 nm in size) were also proposed as a crucial parameter in organ-specific deposition

(Continued)

TABLE 7.2 (Continued)
Nanoparticles for Targeting Different Sites (Yildirimer et al., 2011)

S. No.	Target	Nanocarriers	Characteristics Features
4.	*Brain targets:* because of its limited regenerating ability, it must be protected from external damages. This is accomplished by the protective BBB, which separates the cerebrospinal fluid (CSF) surrounding the brain from systemic blood circulation via tight junctions around capillaries, and is undeniably beneficial in preventing blood-borne pathogens from gaining entry and causing potentially irreversible damage while allowing the diffusion of smaller lipophilic molecules like oxygen. Bypassing the BBB, on the other hand, may be useful and potentially life-saving in the treatment of acute disorders like brain meningitis and chronic illnesses like dementia and Parkinson's disease. Targeted medication delivery allows for lesser therapeutic doses, resulting in fewer systemic side effects	Gold nanoparticles	Larger NPs were discovered to be restricted from accessing cerebral tissues, but ultra-small NPs were shown to be broadly distributed in practically all tissues, including the brain
		Silver nanoparticles	AgNP has been discovered to have neurodegenerative properties. The interaction between AgNP and the BBB has indicated that the BBB is functionally disrupted, resulting in the production of cerebral edema
		Superparamagnetic nanoparticles	The BBB has been functionally disrupted as a result of an interaction between AgNP and BBB, resulting in the production of brain edema SPION is particularly useful for novel therapeutic and diagnostic applications due to its nanoscale size and great surface area to volume ratio. Such dimensional reductions, on the other hand, may cause cytotoxicity and interfere with the cell's natural components and functions
		Quantum dots	Small QDs can move out of the capillary bed and into the brain parenchyma through tiny gaps (20 nm) between astrocytic foot processes that make up the BBB

I. **Oral Administration:** The most prevalent route of drug administration is oral administration, which has a high level of patient acceptability. Because of its ease, pain avoidance, efficacy, high patient compliance, and reduced risk of cross-infection and needle stick injuries, the oral route is the most recommended route for medication administration. The drug's oral availability, on the other hand, is determined by its solubility and permeability. Oral distribution of peptides or proteins is frequently harmed by the gastrointestinal tract's acidic environment and enzymatic system, resulting in protein breakdown and a reduction in therapeutic value. As a result, various critical approaches to improving the stability and absorption of protein and peptide medications have been tested. These include chemical modification of peptides (e.g., lipophilic derivatives and synthesis) and site-specific delivery systems.

Nanotechnology enables (i) the administration of weakly water-soluble medications, (ii) drug targeting to a specific section of the digestive tract, (iii) drug transcytosis through the tight intestinal barrier, and (iv) intracellular and transcellular delivery of big macromolecules. One approach for overcoming the GI barrier, protecting the drug from enzymatic breakdown, and releasing it in a controlled or systemic manner is nanoparticle encapsulation. Another interesting technique to pre-oral delivery of protein and peptide medicines with improved therapeutic efficacy is the use of a biodegradable polymeric nanoparticle. Polymeric nanocarriers can protect pharmaceuticals, improving absorption rates, and the nature of the nanocarrier has a big impact on its stability in the GIT.

Advantages:
- It is the most straightforward, practical, and secure method of drug administration.
- It is practical for frequent and long-term use.
- It is painless and self-administered.
- It is cost-effective because the patient incurs no additional expenses. When taking a solid medicine, such as a tablet or capsule, the patient just requires one or two cups of water, which is usually readily available. If the drug is in liquid form, all that is required is a measuring tool, which is usually included with the drug.
- There are no sterile precautions required.
- The risk of an acute medication reaction is quite low.

Disadvantages:
- Because the start of action of orally taken medications is generally slow, it is not ideal for an emergency.
- It can only be used in people who are awake and able to swallow.
- It necessitates the participation or acquiescence of the patient, particularly in outpatients.
- Unpalatable and extremely irritating medications, pharmaceuticals that are degraded by gastric acid and digestive juices (e.g., insulin), drugs with substantial first-pass metabolism (e.g., lignocaine and imipramine), and patients with severe vomiting and diarrhea are not recommended.

- The oral route of drug administration is occasionally ineffective since absorption is uneven and partial in most situations.

II. **Pulmonary Administration:** In diseases such as COPD, asthma, and cystic fibrosis, the pulmonary or inhalational route of administration has traditionally been employed for drug administration to the respiratory system. A medicine must be in aerosol form, generated by an appropriate instrument, in order to reach the lungs through the bronchial tree. Aerosols are two-phase systems made up of condensed and finely divided materials suspended in a continuous gaseous phase that are reasonably stable. Because of the size constraints imposed by this approach, colloidal dispersion is required, and the dispersed phase can be a liquid (mist), a solid (suspension), or a combination of both.

Although a substantial proportion of researched nanoparticle formulations for inhalation are intended to treat local lung ailments, nanomedicines can be delivered via the pulmonary route for both local and systemic drug administration. Nanomedicines can be used to increase drug solubility and lung deposition kinetics, as well as control drug release in the lungs, in pulmonary drug delivery. Furthermore, nanoparticles have a distinct advantage in pulmonary distribution because their small size prevents them from being taken up by macrophages, which is critical for minimizing drug loss and increasing drug retention and bioavailability. However, if they are supplied as nano-aerosols rather than microparticles, their small size may make them susceptible to exhalation following pulmonary administration. Because the most efficient aerodynamic size range for lung delivery is between 1 and 5 micron, nanomedicine formulation development for pulmonary delivery faces a unique challenge in carefully formulating nanoparticles into an inhalable formulation that can deliver nanoparticles to desired sites in the lungs and exert their effect as nanosystems after inhalation. Following inhalation, the nanoparticles are processed into an inhalable state to achieve uniform lung dispersion, cell-targeted administration, or controlled drug release, among other things (Das et al., 2021).

Inhalation drugs are delivered using one of three devices:
- Inhalers with pressurized canisters that provide predetermined doses by actuating a valve.
- Nebulizers are devices that use either a high-velocity air stream or ultrasonic energy to turn aqueous solutions or suspensions (of micronized medicines) into an aerosol.
- Single-dose and multi-dose dry powder inhalers are available.

    Manufacturing of nanoparticulate inhalation aerosols: Several processing approaches have been applied in the formulation creation of nanoparticles for use as pulmonary inhalation aerosols with desirable properties such as narrow particle size distribution, increased stability, controlled and targeted release, and improved bioavailability. The usual method of producing respirable aerosol particles in the solid form is to jet-mill the medication under nitrogen gas. Respirable aerosol nanoparticles are made using more complex and advanced manufacturing procedures. These respirable particles may be encased in microparticles in the 1–5 micron respirable aerodynamic size range, or the nanoparticles may be tailored to aggregate to a desirable aerodynamic size range. Spray drying (also known as advanced spray drying or nanospray drying), spray-freeze drying, supercritical fluid technology, double emulsion/solvent evaporation technology, antisolvent precipitation, particle replication in nonwetting templates (PRINT), and thermal condensation using capillary aerosol generator are some of the manufacturing nanotechnologies (Mansour et al., 2009).

Advantages: Other advantages of the pulmonary route of drug administration, in addition to fast absorption and beginning of action, include the following:

- There will be fewer systemic negative effects.
- The dose can be removed without contaminating the rest of the container's contents.
- Because labile compounds are better protected from oxygen and moisture breakdown, their stability improves.
- It is possible to administer the medication directly to the affected area in the chosen form.
- Mechanical application produces less or no irritation when compared to topical application.
- The formulation is simple and convenient to use.
- A thin layer of medicine can be administered.
- Protein-based solutions can be inhaled in a nebulizer.
- Drug carriers made of lipid, water, or lipid/water emulsions can be used to alleviate drug solubility difficulties. Viscous medication compositions can also be nebulized this way.
- Patients with respiratory difficulties will benefit from this treatment.
- It is possible to titrate the dose.

Disadvantages:

- Drug delivery to the location of action is not guaranteed.
- Drug irritation and toxicity are possible side effects.
- It's possible that drug retention and clearance will be an issue.
- In vivo, the drug may not be stable.
- It's debatable whether targeting specificity is a good idea.
- The most addictive path (drug can enter the brain quickly).
- It's possible that the patient will have trouble controlling his or her dose.
- Inhalers may be challenging to use for some patients.

III. **Topical Administration:** The application of medication to the surface of the skin or mucous membrane of the eye, ear, nose, mouth, vagina, and other mucous membranes with the goal of limiting the drug's pharmacological effect to the surface or within the layers of skin or mucous membrane is known as the topical route of drug administration. Creams, ointments, gels, lotions, sprays, powders, aerosols, liniments, and drops are the most common topical medications. The topical mode of administration allows for a high local concentration of the medicine to be achieved without disrupting the overall circulation. Absorption into the systemic circulation, on the other hand, is highly prevalent and can have negative consequences. This systemic absorption is sometimes used for medicinal purposes. Topical and/or transdermal drug delivery nanoparticles that are most typically employed.

Nanoparticle-based medication formulations may be tailored for (i) drug retention on the skin surface with no penetration beyond; (ii) drug accumulation inside various layers of the skin where the illness is localized, such as skin neoplasias, depending on the indication. The formulation and medicine would be held for long periods of time with no additional penetration; and (iii) transdermal administration for systemic circulation, where the formulation and drug must penetrate considerably deeper and flow into the bloodstream to treat disorders at remote locations (Krishnan and colleagues, 2020).

Advantages:
- Useful for local delivery of agents, especially those that would be harmful if given systemically.
- Most dermatologic and ophthalmologic treatments contain this ingredient.
- First-pass metabolism is avoided.
- It's simple to use and apply.
- Incompatibility with the gastrointestinal tract will be prevented.
- Avoiding the hazards and difficulties of administration, as well as the many conditions of absorption, such as pH fluctuations, the presence of enzymes, and the time it takes for the stomach to empty, via enteral or parenteral routes.
- Medication discontinuation is simple when necessary.
- Drug is provided to a certain location.
- Drugs with a short biological half-life and a restricted therapeutic window can be used.
- Patient compliance is improved.
- Self-medication is possible.
- Prevents drug levels and hazards from fluctuating.
- Effectiveness is achieved at low doses and with constant drug input.
- In comparison to other routes, this one has a wide range of applications.
- Physiological and pharmacological responses have improved.

Disadvantages:
- Because most medications have a large molecular weight and are lipid insoluble, they cannot be absorbed through the skin or mucous membranes.
- Local skin irritation at the application site is a possibility.
- Some drugs and/or excipients can cause contact dermatitis.
- Can only be used for medications that require a low plasma concentration to work.
- The medications may be denatured by enzymes in the epidermis (Table 7.3).

TABLE 7.3

Merits and Demerits of Different Routes of Administration of Nanoparticles

Oral		Transdermal		Pulmonary		Intravenous	
Advantages	**Limitations**	**Advantages**	**Limitations**	**Advantages**	**Limitations**	**Advantages**	**Limitations**
Non-invasive means of drug delivery	First pass in the metabolism in the liver potentially toxic	Non-invasive means for NP delivery	Local irritation	Non-invasive means for NP delivery	Local toxicity	Systemic delivery of NP	First pass in the metabolism in the liver potentially toxic
	Potential for translocation into systemic circulation	Large surface area	Potential for translocation into systemic circulation	Large surface area	Potential for translocation into systemic circulation	Systemic action	
	Requires intact intestinal mucosa for NP uptake	Local action		Avoiding first-pass metabolism in the liver			

7.3   CONCLUSION

A successful drug delivery to the target region necessitates not only an appropriate nanocarrier but also an effective drug administration method that allows the drug to penetrate the blood–brain barrier. When it comes to targeted drug delivery, however, each route of administration offers advantages and downsides. To overcome the limits of various administration routes, a better understanding of intercellular, transcellular, and other carrier-mediated transportation pathways is required for the next generation of futuristic nanocarriers to be developed. The development of such a sophisticated nanotherapeutic system heralds a new era in nanotechnology-based drug delivery.

REFERENCES

Das, S.C., Khadka, P., Shah, R., McGill, S., & Smyth, H.D.C. (2021). Nanomedicine in pulmonary delivery. *Theory and Applications of Nonparenteral Nanomedicines*, 319–354. https://doi:10.1016/b978-0-12-820466-5.00014-4.

Koppa Raghu, P., Bansal, K.K., Thakor, P., Bhavana, V., Madan, J., Rosenholm, J.M., & Mehra, N.K. (2020). Evolution of nanotechnology in delivering drugs to eyes, skin and wounds via topical route. *Pharmaceuticals*, 13(8), 167. https://doi.org/10.3390/ph13080167.

Mansour, H.M., Rhee, Y.S., & Wu, X. (2009). Nanomedicine in pulmonary delivery. *International Journal of Nanomedicine*, 4, 299–319. https://doi.org/10.2147/ijn.s4937.

Raj, G. Marshall, & Raveendran, R. (2019) Introduction to Basics of Pharmacology and Toxicology: Volume 1: General and Molecular Pharmacology: Principles of Drug Action. 1st edition.

Talevi, A. & Quiroga, P. (2018). ADME Processes in Pharmaceutical Sciences: Dosage, Design, and Pharmacotherapy Success. Switzerland AG: Springer.

Yildirimer, L., Thanh, N., Loizidou, M., & Seifalian, A. (2011). Toxicology and clinical potential of nanoparticles. *Nano Today*, 6, 585–607. https://doi.org/10.1016/j.nantod.2011.10.001.

8 Nanomedicine Approved by FDA and EMEA

8.1 INTRODUCTION

Despite the excitement around the developing subject of nanomedicine, there is still a scarcity of supervision in this field. Most nanomedicines function by interacting directly with genetic materials or with biomolecules essential for normal genome function and cell division, all of which can cause genotoxicity and mutagenicity. The inflammatory response of neutrophils and macrophages causes the formation of reactive oxygen and nitrogen species, which causes oxidative and nitrosative stress. The accumulation of such free radicals in the body can cause substantial damage. This damage can occur in various ways, inducing oxidative DNA damage that leads to strand breakage, protein denaturation and lipid peroxidation that causes cancer, damage to mitochondrial membranes that leads to cell death and necrosis, and transcription of genes involved in carcinogenesis and fibrosis. A variety of data show an accumulation of these particles inside the liver and transfer to sites such as the central nervous, cardiovascular, and renal systems when supplied intravenously. There are too many unknowns that may represent potential hazards to safety for particles that cannot trace after administration. Nanomedicine's precise interactions with biological systems are not yet fully understood, making comprehending, recognizing, and drawing inferences regarding their physicochemical and toxicological features problematic. However, not much is likely to change without standardized regulatory advice in this area. It should also be noted that "one-size" does not fit all in this process, as the unique properties observed at the nanoscale are highly dependent on nanoparticle type, surface properties, administration route, and most importantly, nanoparticle morphology, which can be diverse – something that is indeed slowing down the regulatory process. The regulatory agencies are correct to be cautious; in the past, market permission was required for nanoparticles used in medical imaging, only to be revoked later. The European Medicines Agency (EMA) refused a recommendation for marketing authorization for Sincrem®, an ultra-small superparamagnetic iron oxide (USPIO) contrast agent for magnetic resonance imaging and pulled it from the market in 2008 due to issues identified in clinical trials. These concerns included significant adverse reactions involving muscle pains, notably in the lower back, and allergic reactions that resulted in one death. As a result, the hazards associated with this specific nano molecule greatly outweighed any potential advantages, and it was denied marketing authorization. However, this overly cautious approach appears to be causing significant stagnation within the sector, as the benchmark checks required for approval are frequently opaque and align with the rules for tiny medicinal compounds, which do not require clearance.

- **Regulatory Agencies for Nanomedicines**

    Regulatory agencies such as the FDA employ safety data based on bulk materials, which do not exhibit the same pharmacologic and pharmacokinetic activity as nanomedicines, arguably the most significant obstacle to the regulation of nanomedicines. This means that data generated on safety and efficacy will not be typical of what might happen when nanomedicine is utilized in clinical settings once it has received marketing approval. This complicates the development of laws governing nanomedicines' safety and efficacy criteria because a non-nano version may meet regulatory standards, but a nanomedicine may not. Another significant problem has been encountered in the categorization of nanomedicine. They could be categorized as either medicine or medical equipment, and the classification is not always uniform globally (Foulkes et al., 2020) (Figure 8.1).

- **Challenges in the Development of Pharmaceutical Nanomedicines (Halwani et al., 2022)**

    Over the last 20 years, the field of pharmaceutical nanotechnology has seen tremendous growth and progress. The field of nanomedicine has received particular attention because it has the potential to transform medical care by providing more efficient, less toxic, and intelligent therapies that can be targeted to the location of sickness. Many nanomedicines have been successfully produced and approved for clinical use with a tremendous effort from academia and the biopharmaceutical industry. However, as numerous sorts of problems are encountered during the creation of pharmaceutical nanomedicines, the field of nanomedicine is still in its infancy with few success stories. These difficulties are as follows (Figure 8.2).

- **Developmental Nanomedicines**

    Nanomedicine-based pharmaceutical products are anticipated to play a significant role in the global pharmaceutical marketplace and healthcare system. Since 1995, around 70 nanomedicine products have been permitted by the Food and Drug Administration (FDA) and the European Medicines Agency (EMA) for marketing, and twofold this number are existing in clinical trials. However, most nanomedicines approved to date have revealed reduced toxicity rather than improved efficacy. Many nanoparticle-based drugs have entered the market and are used daily by many patients (Table 8.2). These products come from a variety of companies all over the world and demonstrate the accomplishment of nanomedicines as therapeutic agents. Since 1989, 78 nanomedicines have been approved and are now available on the global market. Of these, 66 nanomedicines have been permitted by the FDA, while 31 nanomedicines have been accepted by the EMA. Twenty nanomedicines have received global approval from both the FDA and the EMA, while other nanomedicines have received approval from only one of the two agencies (FDA: 43 nanomedicines; EMA: 12 nanomedicines). Since 2010, the focus on developing nanomedicines and the number of marketed nanomedicines have significantly increased due to the resulting healthcare system benefits. The globally marketed nanomedicines can be classified

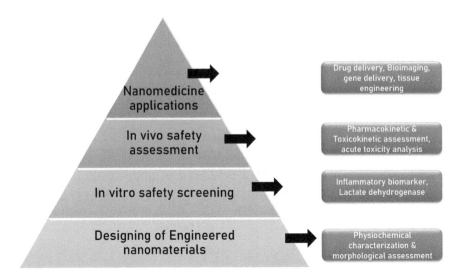

FIGURE 8.1 Pyramid model on the determination of ENMs design, production, and toxicity assessment.

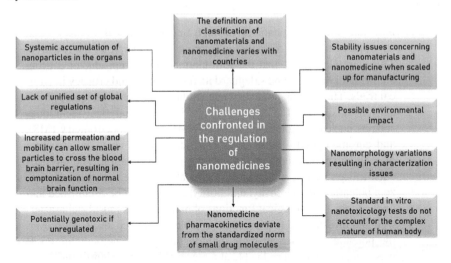

FIGURE 8.2 Diagram highlighting the significant challenges faced in the regulation of nanomaterials (Foulkes et al., 2020).

as nanocrystals, lipid-based nanoparticles, polymer-based nanoparticles, dendrimer-based nanoparticles, protein-based nanoparticles, or inorganic nanoparticles (Halwani and Abdulrahman, 2022).

- **Considerations in Nanomedicine Development (Figure 8.3)**
  i. **Chemistry, Manufacturing, and Controls (CMC) Considerations:** Nanomedicines are more complex than conventional drugs, as they face CMC challenges during product development and in the later stage of manufacturing scale-up. Thus, the first step in developing nanomedicine

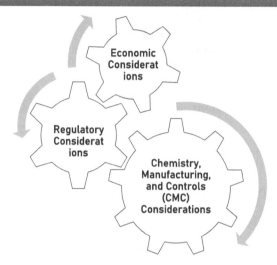

FIGURE 8.3   Major aspects to be considered for developing of a nanomedicine.

is to determine practicability through understanding the makeup and structure of the early formulation to prove the principle in the research. This step will ensure that the formulation can be reproducible during confirmatory studies and safeguard its future safety and efficacy in clinical trials. The early nanomedicine candidates must have adequate physical, chemical, and functional characterization. Analytical techniques such as nuclear magnetic resonance (NMR), mass spectrometry (MS), and chromatography must be used to identify the chemical structure of each component involved in nanoparticle formulation. The physicochemical properties of the early formulated sample, i.e., particle size, zeta potential, pH, viscosity, and purity, also need to be established and understood. The biological functions of nanoparticles must be characterized and investigated to provide acceptable confidence levels. Moreover, the potential commercial-scale manufacturing of nanomedicine products that are easily reproducible at a reasonable cost is significant.

For this reason, the CMC developers should understand the early stages of nanomedicine synthesis and assess whether the chemicals and the processing can be used and performed on an industrial scale. Cytotoxic compounds and complex processing may be achievable on a laboratory scale but may be expensive and challenging on an industrial scale. The manufacturing process of nanomedicines is quite complex, so minimizing the batch-to-batch variability of nanomedicine formulations is a significant challenge. Thus, the quality of the product, which impacts the strength, purity, safety, and efficacy of nanomedicines, is essential for successful development and commercialization.

ii. **Economic Considerations:** It is necessary to ponder over the amount of investment essential to endowment for the expansion of nanomedicine production. The complete risk of CMC development must be well thought out in investment profiles used to compare potential nanomedicine programs to other development portfolios. Instruments, manufacturing equipment, and other facilities may be costlier for some companies; therefore, these facilities must be included in nanomedicine development investment tactics that are associated with clinical necessities.

iii. **Regulatory Considerations:** Early FDA consultations regarding nanomedicine development will help in understanding the scientific and regulatory issues relevant to the product and in addressing questions concerning the safety, effectiveness, public health impact, and regulatory status of the product. Therefore, nanomedicine development should follow the usual pathways and processes of drug development using a suitable evaluation framework. In Europe, the EMA has established an Expert Working Group and has released some reflection papers for particular nanomedicines to guide developers in preparing marketing authorization applications. However, it is not clear whether the existing regulatory frameworks will pose challenges in the future for more innovative nanotechnology.

• **Global Regulatory Agencies**

Some of the major regulatory organizations worldwide are mentioned in Figure 8.4. However, in this chapter, nanomedicines approved by FDA and EMEA are focused.

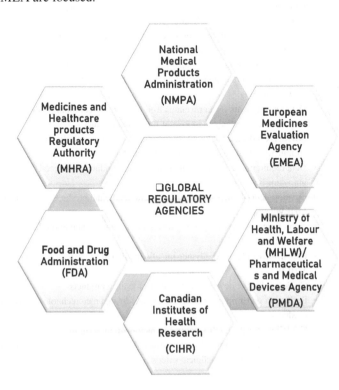

FIGURE 8.4 Major regulatory organizations worldwide.

- **Nanomedicine Guidelines**

  Over the last few decades, approximately 100 nanomedicines and 11 nanomedicines have been approved by the FDA and EMA, respectively, while 48 nanomedicines are presently under clinical trials in the European Union. Considering the increasing number of nanomedicine applications and sharing the experience of the regulatory network in the scientific evaluation of nanomedicines, several guidelines about nanomaterial and nanoproducts were released by the FDA, EMA, Ministry of Health, Labour and Welfare, Japan (MHLW), and Chinese National Medical Products Administration (NMPA). These guidelines involve different nano-dosage forms, including liposomes, iron-based nano-colloidal products, block copolymer micelles, and nucleic acid (siRNA)-loaded nanoproducts. Among these guidelines, all four regulatory agencies guided liposomes, which might be attributed to the relatively common dosage form, and the large numbers approved in market and clinical trials (Liu et al., 2022) (Table 8.1).

TABLE 8.1
Nanomedicine Guidelines Laid by Various Regulatory Agencies

Regulatory Agencies	Guidelines for Nanomedicine
FDA	• **Guidance for Industry:** Considering whether an FDA-regulated creation involves the application of nanotechnology • Drug products, including biological products, that contain nanomaterials guidance for industry (draft) • **Guidance for Industry:** Liposome drug products chemistry, manufacturing, and controls; human pharmacokinetics and bioavailability; and labeling documentation
EMA	• Data requirements for intravenous iron-based nano-colloidal products developed concerning an innovator medicinal product • **Surface Coatings:** General issues for consideration regarding parenteral administration of coated nanomedicine products • Data requirements for intravenous liposomal products developed regarding an innovator liposomal product • Development of block-copolymer-micelle medicinal products – Joint EMA and MHLW • Non-clinical studies for generic nanoparticle iron medicinal product applications
MHLW	• Expansion of block-copolymer-micelle medicinal products – Joint EMA and MHLW • Guideline for the development of liposome drug products • Reflection paper on nucleic acids (siRNA)-loaded nanotechnology-based drug products
NMPA	• Guidelines for the quality control of nanomedicines (draft) • Guidelines for the non-clinical pharmacokinetics of nanomedicines (draft) • Guidelines for the non-clinical safety evaluation of nanomedicines (draft)

TABLE 8.2

List of Globally Marketed Nanomedicines Approved by the FDA and the EMA (Halwani and Abdulrahman, 2022)

Type	Trade Name	Company	Date of Approval	Active Ingredients	Indication
Lipid-based nanoparticles	Abelcet®	Defiante Farmaceutica	FDA (1995)	Amphotericin B	Fungicidal drug
	Doxil®	Johnson & Johnson	FDA (1995), EMA (1996)	Doxorubicin (adriamycin)	Metastatic ovarian cancer, HIV-associated Kaposi's sarcoma (KS)
	DaunoXome®	Galen Ltd	FDA, EMA (1996)	Daunorubicin	Cancers and HIV-associated KS
	Caelyx®	Janssen Pharmaceuticals	EMA (1996)	Doxorubicin	For breast and ovarian cancer, HIV-associated KS
	AmBisome®	NeXstar Pharmaceuticals	EMA (1990), FDA (1997)	Amphotericin B	Fungicidal drug
	Inflexal®	Crucell Berna Biotech	EMA (1997)	Inactivated influenza virus vaccine	For prevention of influenza infection
	Curosurf®	Chiesi	FDA (1999)	Poractant alfa	For respiratory distress syndrome (RDS)
	Myocet®	Teva Pharmaceutical Industries Ltd.	EMA (2000)	Doxorubicin hydrochloride	For breast cancer
	Visudyne®	QLT Phototherapeutics	FDA & EMA (2000)	Photosensitizer (PS), benzoporphyrin	For neovascularization triggered by wet age-associated macular degeneration
	Zevalin®	Bayer Pharma	FDA (2002) Disc.[a] EMA (2004)	^{90}Y-ibritumomab tiuxetan	Lymphoma
	DepoCyt®	Pacira Pharmaceuticals	EMA (2002), FDA (2007)	Cytarabine	For lymphomatous meningitis
	DepoDur®	Skye Pharma	FDA (2004), EMA (2006)	Liposomal morphine sulfate	Post-operative analgesics
	Mepact®	Takeda France SAS	EMA (2009)	Mifamurtide	For osteogenic sarcoma

(Continued)

TABLE 8.2 (Continued)

List of Globally Marketed Nanomedicines Approved by the FDA and the EMA (Halwani and Abdulrahman, 2022)

Type	Trade Name	Company	Date of Approval	Active Ingredients	Indication
	Marqibo®	Talon Therapeutics	FDA (2012)	Vincristine	For Philadelphia chromosome-negative chronic myelogenous leukemia in grown-up patients
	Lipodox®	Sun Pharma Global FZE	FDA (2013)	Doxorubicin hydrochloride	HIV-associated KS and metastatic ovarian cancer
	Onivyde®	Merrimack Pharmaceuticals	FDA (2015)	Irinotecan	For metastatic cancer of pancreas
	Lipusu®	Jazz Pharmaceutics	FDA (2016)	Paclitaxel	For non-small cell lung cancer (NSCLC) and cancer of the breast
	Vyxeos®	Jazz Pharmaceutics	FDA (2017), EMA (2018)		For acute myeloid leukemia
	Onpattro®	Alnylam	FDA & EMA (2018)	Patisiran	For hereditary transthyretin (TTR)-mediated amyloidosis
	Pfizer-BioNTech Vaccine	Pfizer Pharmaceuticals	FDA (2020)	mRNA vaccine	For prevention of COVID-19 infection
	Moderna COVID-19 Vaccine	ModernaTX Inc.	FDA (2020)	mRNA vaccine	For prevention of COVID-19 infection
Polymer-based nanoparticles	Diprivan®	Fresenius Kabi	FDA (1989), EMA (2001)	Propofol	(Sedative-hypnotic agent) to induce relaxation before and during general anesthesia used during surgery
	Adagen®	Enzon Pharmaceuticals Inc.	FDA (1990)	Adenosine deaminase (ADA)	To be used in adenosine deaminase (ADA)-severe combined immunodeficiency disorder
	Renagel®	Sanofi	FDA (2000)	Sevelamer carbonate	For hyperphosphatemia instigated by chronic kidney disease (CKD)

(Continued)

TABLE 8.2 (Continued)
List of Globally Marketed Nanomedicines Approved by the FDA and the EMA (Halwani and Abdulrahman, 2022)

Type	Trade Name	Company	Date of Approval	Active Ingredients	Indication
	PegIntron®	Merk & Co. Inc.	EMA (2000), FDA (2001)	Alpha interferon (INF) molecule	Used in hepatitis C
	Eligard®	Tolmar Pharmaceuticals Inc.	FDA (2002)	Leuprolide acetate	For prostate cancer
	Neulasta®	Amgen, Inc.	FDA (2002)	Filgrastim	Febrile neutropenia; resulting infections arising due to deficiency of neutrophils
	Pegasys®	Genentech USA, Inc	FDA, EMA (2002)	Recombinant human alfa-2a interferon	For hepatitis B and hepatitis C
	Somavert®	Pfizer Pharmaceuticals	EMA (2002), FDA (2003)	Analog of human growth hormone (acts as an antagonist of G.H. receptors)	To be used in acromegaly
	Restasis®	Allergan	FDA (2003)	Cyclosporine	To be used in chronic dry eye
	Estrasorb™	Novavax, Inc.	FDA (2003)	Hemihydrate	Moderate vasomotor symptoms due to menopause
	Macugen®	Pfizer Pharmaceuticals	FDA (2004)	Pegaptinib sodium	Choroidal neovascularization caused by wet age-related macular degeneration
	Genexol-PM®	Lupin Ltd.	FDA (2007)	Paclitaxel	Breast cancer
	Renagel®/Renvela®	Genzyme	EMA (2007)	Sevelamer HCL	Hyperphosphatemia caused by CKD
	Krystexxa®	Savient Pharmaceuticals	FDA (2010)	Pegloticase is a recombinant porcine-like uricase	For chronic refractory gout
	Plegridy®	Biogen	FDA (2014)	Recombinant IFN-β	For remitting multiple sclerosis (RRMS) relapsing in adult patients
	Adynovate®	Baxalta US Inc.	FDA (2015)	Coagulation factor VIII	Hemophilia A

(Continued)

TABLE 8.2 (Continued)

List of Globally Marketed Nanomedicines Approved by the FDA and the EMA (Halwani and Abdulrahman, 2022)

Type	Trade Name	Company	Date of Approval	Active Ingredients	Indication
	Copaxone®/FOGA	Teva Pharmaceutical Industries Ltd.	FDA (1996), EMA (2016)	Glatiramer acetate	Multiple sclerosis (MS)
	Oncaspar®	Enzon Pharmaceuticals Inc.	FDA (1994), EMA (2016)	L-asparaginase	For acute lymphoblastic leukemia and chronic myelogenous leukemia
	Rebinyn®	Novo Nordisk	FDA (2017)	Recombinant DNA-derived coagulation FIX	Hemophilia B
	Zilretta®	Flexion Therapeutics	FDA (2017)	Triamcinolone acetonide	For knee osteoarthritis
	Apealea®	Oasmia Pharmaceutical AB	EMA (2018)	Paclitaxel	For peritoneal and ovarian cancer
	Mircera®	Vifor	EMA (2007), FDA (2018)	Epoetin β (EPO) (EPO is a genetically recombinant form of erythropoietin)	To be used in anemia
Dendrimer based nanoparticles	VivaGel®	BV Starpharma	FDA (2015)	Astodrimer sodium	Effective for prevention of recurrent bacterial vaginosis (BV)
Inorganic nanoparticles	Infed®	Actavis Pharma	FDA (1992)	Iron dextran	For iron deficiency in CKD
	Dexferrum®	American Regent	FDA (1996)	Iron dextran	For iron deficiency in CKD
	Venofer®	Luitpold Pharm	FDA (2000)	Iron sucrose	For iron deficiency in CKD
	GastroMARK™/Umirem®	Mallinckrodt Inc.	FDA (2009) Disc.[a] 2012	SPION-silicone	Used as imaging agent
	Feridex®/Endorem®	AMAG Pharma	FDA (1996) Disc.[a] 2008	SPION-dex	Used as imaging agent
	Feraheme™	AMAG Pharmaceuticals	FDA (2009)	Ferumoxytol	To be used in anemia

(Continued)

TABLE 8.2 (Continued)
List of Globally Marketed Nanomedicines Approved by the FDA and the EMA (Halwani and Abdulrahman, 2022)

Type	Trade Name	Company	Date of Approval	Active Ingredients	Indication
	Ferrlecit®	Sanofi-Aventis	FDA (1999), EMA (2013)	Sodium ferric gluconate	For iron deficiency in CKD
	Ferinject®	Vifor	FDA, EMA (2013)	Iron carboxymaltose colloid	For iron deficient anemia
	Hensify®	Nanobiotix	EMA (2019)	Hafnium oxide nanoparticles	Effective against locally advanced squamous cell carcinoma
Protein-based nanoparticles	Ontak®	Eisai	FDA (1999)	Diphtheria toxin	For leukemia and T-cell lymphoma
	Abraxane®	Celgene Pharmaceutical Co. Ltd.	FDA (2005, 2012, 2013), EMA (2008)	Paclitaxel	Approved by the FDA for treatment of metastatic breast, lung cancer, and metastatic pancreatic adenocarcinoma
Nanocrystals	TriCor®	Abbott Laboratories	FDA (2004)	Fenofibrate	Antihyperlipidemic

a Discontinued.

8.2   CONCLUSION

The increasing research in nanomedicine has aided in the reformulation of existing medicines as well as the development of new ones. Some of the modifications introduced by nanotechnology in medicines include changes in toxicity, solubility, and bioavailability profile. In order to approve new and innovative nanomedicines in the pharmaceutical market, guidelines for the development and evaluation of nanomedicines must be developed in order for different stakeholders to have a common understanding. This process must be carried out in tandem with interagency harmonization efforts in order to support rational decisions on scientific and regulatory issues, financing, and market admittance.

REFERENCES

Foulkes, R., Man, E., Thind, J., Yeung, S., Joy, A., & Hoskins, C. (2020). The regulation of nanomaterials and nanomedicines for clinical application: current and future perspectives. *Biomaterials Science*, 8(17), 4653–4664. https://doi.org/10.1039/d0bm00558d.
Halwani, A.A. (2022). Development of pharmaceutical nanomedicines: from the bench to the market. *Pharmaceutics*, 14, 106. https://doi.org/10.3390/ pharmaceutics14010106.
Liu, P., Chen, G., & Zhang, J. (2022). A review of liposomes as a drug delivery system: current status of approved products, regulatory environments, and future perspectives. *Molecules*, 27(4), 1372. https://doi.org/10.3390/molecules27041372.
Soares, S., Sousa, J., Pais, A., & Vitorino, C. (2018). Nanomedicine: principles, properties, and regulatory issues. *Frontiers in Chemistry*, 6. https://doi:10.3389/fchem.2018.00360.

9 Nanoparticulate Carriers Used as Vaccine Adjuvant Delivery Systems

9.1 INTRODUCTION

Classical vaccines contain live attenuated microbes, killed microbes, or microbe elements. Although many of these vaccines have been critical in the control of infectious disease, some do not provide adequate disease protection. Furthermore, some live vaccines are not safe for use in society's growing population of immuno-compromised people. There are also a number of infectious diseases for which there are no licensed vaccines. To address these issues, a variety of vaccines based on isolated proteins, polysaccharides, or naked DNA encoding a protective antigen are being developed. While these vaccines may be safer, more defined, and less reactogenic than many existing vaccines, they are frequently poor immunogens that require adjuvants to improve their efficacy. Adjuvants based on aluminum are the most commonly used ones, but they can cause local reactions and may fail to generate strong cell-mediated immunity. As a result, there is a significant need for novel adjuvants and delivery systems for the next generation of vaccines.

Adjuvants are compounds that, when combined with vaccine antigens, induce a stronger and more efficacious response to the vaccine than the vaccine alone. Adjuvants have been added to vaccines to (i) improve the immunogenicity of antigens; (ii) reduce the amount of antigen or the number of immunizations required for protective immunity; and (iii) improve vaccine efficacy in newborns, the elderly, and immunocompromised people.

Adjuvants are broadly classified into two types: immunostimulatory adjuvants and vaccine delivery systems.

- Immunostimulatory adjuvants (immunopotentiators) are derived from pathogens, and they represent pathogen-associated molecular patterns (PAMPs) (e.g., lipopolysaccharide (LPS), monophosphoryl lipid (MPL), cytosine phosphor guanine deoxynucleotides (CpG DNA)) and initiate innate immunity directly (via cytokines) or pattern recognition receptors (PRRs).
- Vaccine delivery systems concentrate and display antigens, vaccine antigens are targeted to antigen-presenting cells (APCs) and they aid in the co-localization of antigens and immunopotentiators (Figure 9.1).

DOI: 10.1201/9781003252122-9

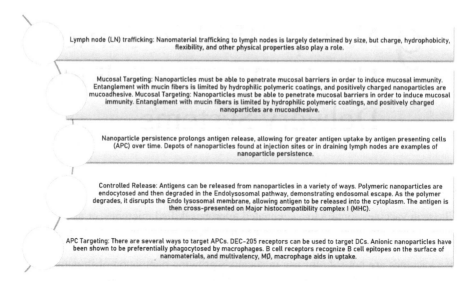

Lymph node (LN) trafficking: Nanomaterial trafficking to lymph nodes is largely determined by size, but charge, hydrophobicity, flexibility, and other physical properties also play a role.

Mucosal Targeting: Nanoparticles must be able to penetrate mucosal barriers in order to induce mucosal immunity. Entanglement with mucin fibers is limited by hydrophilic polymeric coatings, and positively charged nanoparticles are mucoadhesive. Mucosal Targeting: Nanoparticles must be able to penetrate mucosal barriers in order to induce mucosal immunity. Entanglement with mucin fibers is limited by hydrophilic polymeric coatings, and positively charged nanoparticles are mucoadhesive.

Nanoparticle persistence prolongs antigen release, allowing for greater antigen uptake by antigen presenting cells (APC) over time. Depots of nanoparticles found at injection sites or in draining lymph nodes are examples of nanoparticle persistence.

Controlled Release: Antigens can be released from nanoparticles in a variety of ways. Polymeric nanoparticles are endocytosed and then degraded in the Endolysosomal pathway, demonstrating endosomal escape. As the polymer degrades, it disrupts the Endo lysosomal membrane, allowing antigen to be released into the cytoplasm. The antigen is then cross-presented on Major histocompatibility complex I (MHC).

APC Targeting: There are several ways to target APCs. DEC-205 receptors can be used to target DCs. Anionic nanoparticles have been shown to be preferentially phagocytosed by macrophages. B cell receptors recognize B cell epitopes on the surface of nanomaterials, and multivalency, MØ, macrophage aids in uptake.

FIGURE 9.1   Strategies for engineering nanomaterial vaccine delivery (Fries et al. 2021).

9.2   RATIONAL DESIGN OF VACCINE ADJUVANTS

Pathogen vaccinology determines the appropriate immune responses, which are then defined by the sort of vaccine; distinct immune responses may be required for a prophylactic vaccine that prevents disease and a therapeutic vaccine that treats disease or prevents clinical signs. The relevant innate immune cells must be identified based on the required immune responses, as well as their localization within the body and PRR expression on target cells. These factors can be used to develop the delivery system as well as identify relevant immunostimulatory molecules. The delivery systems are usually nanoparticle-based structures of various origins, such as liposomes, emulsions, virosomes, or aluminum salts. The design of delivery systems is influenced by factors such as the site of the target innate cells, the route of administration, the immunostimulators used, and the mode of antigen association. The PRR expression of target innate cell subsets is frequently used to determine the important immunostimulators. These could be APCs (e.g., dendritic cells and macrophages) or cells with bystander function. Independent of adjuvant design programs, antigen discovery programs can identify immunogenic antigens for a given pathogen and use them to develop recombinant antigens that, when combined with appropriate adjuvants, induce pathogen-specific immune responses. In relevant animal models, the vaccine formulation (adjuvant + antigen) is tested in vivo to characterize the induced

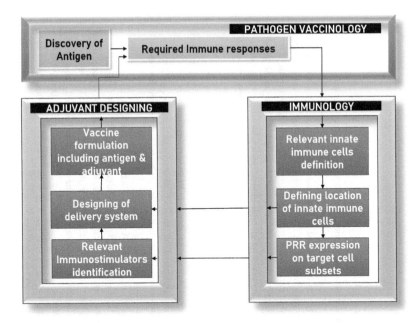

FIGURE 9.2 Rational designing of vaccine adjuvants.

immune responses, and possibly, the action to a pathogen issue (Schmidt et al. 2018) (Figure 9.2).

9.3 NANOPARTICLES AS VACCINE DELIVERY VEHICLES

Recently, there has been increased interest in the use of nanoparticles (NPs) as vaccine carriers. The vaccine antigen is either encapsulated within the NP or embellished on its exterior. NPs, by encapsulating antigenic substance, therefore provide approach for delivering antigens that would otherwise degrade quickly after injection or elicit a short-lived, localized immune response. Conjugation of antigens onto NPs can allow the immunogen to be presented to immune systems in the same way as that of the pathogen, eliciting a similar response. Furthermore, NPs made from some composites enable not only site-directed antigen delivery but also prolonged antigen release to maximize immune system exposure. The propensity for NPs to deliver vaccines via non-traditional approaches such as topical, inhalation, or optical delivery, as well as combining multiple antigens to the same particle to protect against more than one disease, is also being investigated (Gregory et al. 2013) (Tables 9.1–9.3).

TABLE 9.1

Categories of Nanoparticles as Vaccines Adjuvants (Petkar et al. 2021)

Nanoparticles Classes	Description
Viral vectored vaccines	A viral vector is a naturally evolved (from virus) vehicle that is a valuable technique for introducing genetic material into the host cell for gene delivery and vaccines to initiate immune responses. Because of their unique properties such as encapsulation and protection of sensitive compounds, ease of exterior modification, innate biocompatibility, and naturally immunogenicity, viral vectors have played an important role in the development of vaccines, leading to their development as actively targeted drug delivery systems. Because of their ability to elicit a robust immune response, viral vectors such as retrovirus, lentivirus, adenovirus, adeno-associated virus, herpesvirus, poxvirus, vesicular stomatitis virus, alphavirus, measles virus, poliovirus, cytomegalovirus, Sendai virus, and HBV have been used in clinical/preclinical trials. Every viral vector has distinct advantages such as genome stability, ease of production, cost-effectiveness, cell specificity over live/attenuated vaccines, ability to deliver multiple immunogenic with efficient expression and strong immune response, long-term gene expression, infects non-dividing and dividing cells, high immunogenicity, induction of unique cytotoxic T lymphocyte (CTL) response, while disadvantages include low titer production, generation of replication-competent virus, the potential for tumorigenesis, ability to infect only dividing cells
Virus-like particles (VLPs) and virosomes	VLPs are empty, multiprotein, non-replicating and non-infectious structures resembling natural virions, which are prepared spontaneously during in vitro protein expression by the self-assembly mechanism of viral protein. Subunit vaccine (delivery system) similar to VLPs is called virosomes, which contains an envelope of mono- or bilayer phospholipid vesicles to which additional components of the virus or pathogen/antigen and virus-derived proteins may be attached or inserted. Promising characteristics of VLPs and virosomes resulted in many marketed products (e.g., hepatitis B virus (HBV), human papilloma virus) and fruitful studies under different phases of clinical trials
Non-viral vectors	Non-viral vectors are often called delivery vehicles and typically consist of DNA (usually plasmid DNA produced in bacteria) or RNA as an antigen which is delivered to the target cell to elicit immune response. In addition to nucleic acids, protein and peptide antigens delivery by non-viral vectors also shows great potential in vaccine development. However, the potential drawbacks of endonuclease degradation, lower efficiency, and repeated doses of naked DNA vaccine have been reduced using delivery vehicles. Therefore, natural or synthetic materials (lipids, polymers) have been utilized to prepare non-viral vectors which encapsulate or adsorb antigen and fuse with the cell membrane to release it into the cytoplasm of the cell. Vaccination with non-viral vectors presents many advantages over viral vectors like safety and efficacy (due to the absence of viral component), no limit to DNA insert size, ease in large scale production, low or no-host immunogenicity, protection of antigens, targeting, long-lasting gene expression, and adjuvant effect. Some of the widely investigated adjuvants and delivery systems such as adjuvants are discussed below:

(Continued)

TABLE 9.1 (Continued)
Categories of Nanoparticles as Vaccines Adjuvants (Petkar et al. 2021)

Nanoparticles Classes	Description

1. Nanoemulsion-Based Adjuvants

- **MF59** is an oil-in-water (o/w) emulsion. An MF59-adjuvanted seasonal influenza vaccine (Fluad®) was the first MF59 vaccine to be licensed in 1997. MF59 is a superior adjuvant than alum in inducing both antibody and T cell responses for the influenza vaccine, and side effects such as pain at the injection site and reactogenicity have been observed in some patients.

- **Montanide™:** SEPPIC Inc. (Paris, France) developed highly refined emulsifiers from the mannide monooleate family in a natural metabolizable oil solution, which were named as Montanide ISA 50V, 51, ISA 206, 720. Among these, ISA 50V, 51 and 720 are w/o emulsions, while ISA 206 is a water-in-oil-in-water (w/o/w) double emulsion with particle size ranging between 10 and 500nm. Although these adjuvants have been shown to induce a strong immune response, severe local reactions have limited their use. Currently, Montanide adjuvanted vaccines, in particular ISA™51, against many diseases such as malaria, HIV, and various cancers are under different phases of clinical trials

2. Lipid Nanocarriers Immunostimulatory Complexes (ISCOMs): ISCOM adjuvants are particulate complexes containing protein antigen, saponin adjuvant (Quil A which is derived from the bark of the South American Quillaia saponaria Molina tree), cholesterol, and phospholipids. The cholesterol strongly interacts with saponin to form a unique cage-like particulate structure with a size of 40nm, which is likely to contribute to the stability of the adjuvant and also reduces the hemolytic activity of the saponins which is important for its safety. ISCOM complex traps the protein antigens (typically hydrophobic membrane proteins) through apolar interactions. ISCOMs can bind and penetrate cellular membranes and helps deliver the immunogen into the cytosol of the target cell leading to endogenous processing and presentation of the immunogenic peptide. Thus, ISCOMs represent good vehicles for intracellular delivery of DNA-based vaccines

- *Liposomes:* Liposomes are spherical vesicles, with size ≤500nm, composed of amphiphilic phospholipids and cholesterol, which self-associate into bilayers with an aqueous interior that can encapsulate many drug molecules including protein and DNA-based vaccines. In the delivery of vaccines, the antigen (be it peptide, mRNA, or DNA) can either be adsorbed on the surface of the liposome, loaded in the liposome core, or the lipid bilayer. Liposomes enable efficient delivery of mRNA and have been extensively used to deliver both conventional and self-amplifying mRNA against infectious pathogens

- *Biodegradable Polymeric Nanoparticles:* Biodegradable polymeric NPs (PNPs) display interesting features related to the protection/stabilization of vaccine antigens until they reach the target site. A large number of polymers exist from which PNPs can be prepared, among which widely used polymers like poly-(D,L–lactide-co-glycolide) (PLGA), poly(lactic acid) (PLA), poly(alkyl cyanoacrylate) (PACA), polyanhydrides, and chitosan are already approved by the FDA for use in humans (e.g., as sutures, bone implants, and screws as well as implants for sustained drug delivery). The biodegradable properties of these polymers make them promising vehicles for the exploration of antigen delivery

- *Non-Biodegradable Nanoparticles:* Various non-biodegradable materials such as gold, carbon, silica, quantum dots, and polystyrene have been utilized as vaccine delivery systems and adjuvants. They remain in the tissue for an extended period of time and can thus present the antigen to tissues with enhanced immunogenicity. In general, this is achieved by surface functionalization of nanomaterial to target specific cells. Although non-biodegradable materials facilitate conjugation with different functional groups and antigens, they induce higher cellular and humoral response but often lead to toxicity and aggregation in tissues requiring further validation of safety. Gold nanoparticles (GNPs) are efficient adjuvant and delivery vehicles with or without surface functionalization

(Continued)

TABLE 9.1 (Continued)
Categories of Nanoparticles as Vaccines Adjuvants (Petkar et al. 2021)

Nanoparticles Classes	Description
	• *Calcium Phosphate NPs (CPNPs):* For more than 30 years, calcium phosphate has been used to deliver genetic material to mammalian cells. It has good biocompatibility because it is a naturally occurring, easily absorbed normal body constituent, which eliminates safety concerns. It was used in the form of calcium phosphate gel or suspension as an adjuvant in childhood diphtheria–tetanus–pertussis (DTP) vaccine formulations in France until the 1980s. Many such preclinical studies have found that functionalized calcium phosphate nanoparticles (100–400 nm) can induce both innate and adaptive immunity through dendritic cell (DC) activation. According to BioSante Pharmaceuticals, Inc., CPNPs have a better immunostimulatory effect than aluminum (alum) adjuvants for HSV-2 and Epstein–Barr virus (EBV) infections. As an alternative to aluminum, CPNPs are being researched
	• *Colloidally Stable Nanoparticles:* Because of their water solubility, carbohydrates, such as dextran, pullulan, and mannose, cannot self-associate in an aqueous solution. They can be amphiphilic by being conjugated to hydrophobic materials (e.g., cholesterol). The self-assembly of these molecules (both with and without proteins) results in the formation of colloidally stable nanoparticles with sizes ranging from 30 to 40 nm. The substitution degree of hydrophobes and the hydrophobicity can be changed to control the size, density, and colloidal stability of the nanoparticles
	• *Proteosomes:* The proteosome is made up of hydrophobic, proteinaceous nanoparticles (150 nm) made up of *Neisseria meningitidis* major outer membrane proteins (OMPs). Since 1981, OMPs have been used successfully in a marketed meningococcal vaccine (Menomune®, Sanofi Pasteur). Because of the noncovalent relations between the proteosome and the antigen, which results in the formation of appropriate complexes, hydrophobic OMP is an excellent system for the delivery of polar or amphiphilic antigens. Several human clinical trials have proven proteosomes to be safe and well-tolerated materials for human use, primarily following intranasal administration
3. Adjuvants Targeting Pattern Recognition Receptors (PRRs): Pattern recognition receptors (PRRs) are receptors in the immune system that are specialized in their recognition of pathogens. These receptors are essential components of the innate immune system and are primarily expressed by APCs like DCs and macrophages; however, they are also noticed in other immune and non-immune cells. Bacteria, viruses, fungi, and parasites all exhibit conserved sets of molecular patterns known as pathogen-associated molecular patterns (PAMPs). PAMPs are recognized by APCs via membrane-bound and intracellular receptors known as PRRs.	
	• *C-Type Lectin Receptors (CLRs):* CLRs are transmembrane receptors that distinguish carbohydrate structures embodied by various pathogens.
	• *Toll-Like Receptor (TLRs):* TLRs are integral membrane-bound receptors that are required for innate immunity and help shape the adaptive immune response. TLRs are activated by a variety of PAMPs (including LPS) and threat-assisted molecular patterns (DAMPs). PAMPs and DAMPs can activate a variety of TLRs relative positions in the cell and/or availability following pathogen endocytosis or replication. TLRs are regarded as the first line of immune defense in mammals varies, but they all have the same function of activating inflammatory mediators

TABLE 9.2
Overview of the Various Types of NPs Previously Been Studied for Their Use as Vaccine Carriers (Gregory et al., 2013)

	Matrix/Expression System	Loading	Size	Antigen (Pathogen)	Route of Immunization
Virus-like particles	Baculovirus (Sf9, Sf21, Hi5); *E. coli*; Mammalian cells; Yeast	20–80 µg; 50 µg; 10 µg	55–60 nm (HPV); 100–200 nm (HIV); 80–120 nm (H1N1)	Major capsid protein, L1 (HPV); FMS-like tyrosine kinase receptor ligand, FL (HIV); gag precursor protein, pr45 (HIV); HIV env cDNA (HIV); Haemagglutinin (H1N1); Nicotinamide (H1N1) Matrix protein M1 (H1N1)	Intramuscular, Subcutaneous, Intraperitoneal, Oral, Intranasal
Liposomes (non-viral lipids)	Monophosphoryl lipid A (MPLA); Phospholipid S100 and cholesterol; Phosphatidylcholine and cholesterol	1.26 mg/mL; 0.005 mg/mL; 0.8–1 mg/mL; 0.2 mg/mL	50–500 nm	R32NS1 (malaria); Cholera toxin; Circumsporozoite (malaria); Lipid A; CtUBE fusion peptide (*Helicobacter pylori*); KWC *Yersinia pestis*	Intramuscular, Intravenous, Subcutaneous, Oral, Intranasal
ISCOMs	Saponin (Quil A) Phospholipid (phosphatidylethanolamine, phosphatidylcholine) Cholesterol Viral proteins	1–10 µg; 10 µg; 30 µg; 100–500 µg	40 nm	HIV-1 (gp120/160); FIV (p130); *Eucalyptus falciformis* (p27)	Intramuscular, Subcutaneous, Oral
Non-degradable	Gold; Silica; Carbon	1 mg/mL	2–150 nm; 5–470 nm	Plasmid DNA expressing haemagglutinin 1 (Influenza); Hepatitis B	Intradermal, Intramuscular, Subcutaneous, Intravenous
Polymeric	Poly(lactic-co-glycolic acid) (PLGA); Poly(lactic acid) (PLA); Poly(glycolic acid) (PGA); Poly(hydroxybutyrate) (PHB); Chitosan	42.5 mg/mL; 10–50 µg/mL	100–200 nm; 800 nm; 1–5 µm; 248 nm	Docetaxel; TetHc (Tetanus); Hepatitis B; SBm7462 (*Boophilus microplus*); Rv1733c (*Mycobacterium tuberculosis*); SPf66 (*Plasmodium falciparum* malaria); Dtxd (Diphtheria)	Intramuscular, Intravenous

TABLE 9.3

Approved and Clinically Tested Vaccines Using Nanocarrier-Based Adjuvants and Delivery Systems (Petkar et al., 2021)

Product	Application	Adjuvants Used	Approval Year, Company, Status of Research
Viral Vectored Vaccines			
ACAM2000	Smallpox	MVA-BN	2007, Sanofi Pasteur Biologics Co., Cambridge, MA, USA
Chimpanzee adenovirus vector (ChAdOx1)	Severe acute respiratory syndrome coronavirus 2 (SARS-CoV-2), Coronavirus disease (COVID-19)	Chimpanzee Adenoviral vector	2020, University of Oxford in collaboration with AstraZeneca, Cambridge, UK
Sputnik V (Gam-Covid-Vac)	SARS-CoV-2, COVID-19	Replication-deficient Ad types 5 and 26 vectors	2020, Gamaleya Research Institute, Acellena Contract Drug Research and Development, Moscow, Russia
COVISHIELD™ (ChAdOx1)	SARS-CoV-2, COVID-19	Chimpanzee Adenoviral vector	2020, Serum Institute of India Pvt. Ltd., Pune, Maharashtra, India
Convidicea (Ad5nCoV)	SARS-CoV-2, COVID-19	Recombinant Adenoviral vector, Ad5	2020, CanSino Biologics, Tianjin China (approved for use in Mexico, China)
Janssen COVID-19 Vaccine (Ad26)	SARS-CoV-2, COVID-19	Adenoviral vector, Ad 26	2021, Janssen Biotech, Inc., Horsham, PA, USA (Emergency use authorization by US FDA)
Virus Like Particles			
Recombivax HB®	Hepatitis B Virus (HBV)	Amorphous aluminum hydroxyphosphate sulfate	1986, Merck and Co. Inc., Kenilworth, NJ, USA
Engerix-B	HBV	Aluminum hydroxide	1989, GlaxoSmithkline (GSK), Middlesex, UK
Gardasil®	Human papillomavirus (HPV), cervical cancer and genital warts	Hydroxyphosphate sulfate	2006, Merck and Co. Inc., Kenilworth, NJ, USA
Cervarix	HPV	AS04 (aluminum hydroxide and MPLA)	2009, GlaxoSmithkline Biologicals SA, Rixensart, Belgium
Hecolin	Hepatitis E Virus (HEV)	Aluminum hydroxide	2011, Xiamen Innovax Biotech, Xiamen, Fujian, China
Gardasil-9®	HPV	Hydroxyphosphate sulfate	2014, Merck and Co. Inc., Kenilworth, NJ, USA
Heplisav-B	HBV	1018 ISS CpG ODN	2017, Dynavax Technologies Corporation, Emeryville, CA, USA
Sci-B-Vac®	HBV	Aluminum hydroxide	2020 (under regulatory approval process) VBI Vaccines Inc., Cambridge, MA, USA

(Continued)

TABLE 9.3 (*Continued*)
Approved and Clinically Tested Vaccines Using Nanocarrier-Based Adjuvants and Delivery Systems (Petkar et al., 2021)

Product	Application	Adjuvants Used	Approval Year, Company, Status of Research
Mosquirixs	Malaria and HBV	AS01 (MPL and Quillaja saponaria 21 (QS21))	2015, GlaxoSmithKline Biologicals SA, Rixensart, Belgium
Virosome-Based Vaccine			
Epaxal™	Hepatitis A virus (HAV)	IRIV	1994, Berna Biotech Ltd., Berne, Switzerland
Inflexal® V	Influenza vaccine	IRIV	1997, Berna Biotech Ltd., Berne, Switzerland
Invivac®	Influenza vaccine	IRIV	2004, Solvay Pharmaceuticals B.V., DA Weesp, The Netherlands
NasalFlu®	Influenza vaccine	IRIV	2001, Berna Biotech Ltd., Berne, Switzerland
Epaxal Junior™	Novel pandemic A influenza virus (H1N1)	IRIV	1994, Berna Biotech Ltd., Berne, Switzerland
Non-Viral Vectored Vaccines			
Celtura®	H1N1	MF59	2009, Novartis AG, Basel, Switzerland
Fluad®	Seasonal influenza in infants and young children	MF59	1997, Novartis AG, Basel, Switzerland Phase III Trials Completed 2010–11
Aflunov®	Pre-pandemic influenza (H5N1)	MF59	2010, Seqirus S.R.L., Monteriggioni, SI, Italy
Montanide	Malaria, HIV, cancer	MF59	Under clinical trial
FENDRIX	HBV	Aluminum phosphate and MPLA	2005, GlaxoSmithKline Biologicals, Rixensart, Belgium
Stimuvax®	Lung, breast, prostate, and colorectal cancer	Liposome, MPLA	Merck KGaA, Darmstadt, Germany, Phase III Clinical Trial Completed
mRNA-1273	COVID-19	Liposome	2020, Moderna, Cambridge, MA, USA
BNT162b2	COVID-19	Liposome	2020, Pfizer, New York, NY, USA and BioNTech, Mainz, Rhineland-Palatinate, Germany
Prevnar®	Invasive Pneumococcal disease	Aluminum phosphate	2000, Wyeth Pharmaceuticals, Madison, NJ, USA
Menactra®	Meningococcal disease	Aluminum	2005, Sanofi Pasteur, Lyon, France

Abbreviations: SARS-CoV-2, severe acute respiratory syndrome coronavirus 2; COVID-19, coronavirus disease; MVA-BN, modified vaccinia Ankara-BN; ChAdOx1, Chimpanzee adenovirus vector; Ad 26, adenoviral vector; HBV, Hepatitis B Virus; HPV, human papillomavirus; HEV, Hepatitis E Virus; IRIV, immunopotentiating reconstituted influenza virosome; H1N1, novel pandemic A influenza virus; H5N1, pre-pandemic influenza; MPLA, monophosphoryl lipid A; CpG ODN, cytosine-phosphorothioate-guanine oligodeoxynucleotides; IRIV, immunopotentiating reconstituted influenza virosome; MVA-BN, Modified Vaccinia Ankara-Bavarian Nordic.

9.4 CONCLUSION

A number of NP-based VADSs are currently in development. Many of them have demonstrated the ability to decentralized approach antigens (Ag) via different vaccination trails in order to garner anti-Ag immunity at the systemic and even mucosal stages, thereby offering additional recipes for vaccines targeting infectious pathogens and even cancers. Certain NP-based VADSs with multiple advantages, such as specific targeting, diverse modification, good biocompatibility, and high Ag delivery efficiency, have brought a few subunit vaccines to market for clinical vaccination, which is encouraging. Many of the issues associated with the development of NP VADSs, such as safety; availability; production scale-up; and the cost of synthetic materials, functional molecules, and whole products, will undoubtedly be resolved, and more NP-based VADS will be approved for clinical use, providing opportunities to conquer.

REFERENCES

Fries, C. N., Curvino, E. J., Chen, J.-L., Permar, S. R., Fouda, G. G., & Collier, J. H. (2020). Advances in nanomaterial vaccine strategies to address infectious diseases impacting global health. *Nature Nanotechnology*, 8, e61135. https://doi.org/10.1038/s41565-020-0739-9.

Gregory, A. E., Titball, R., & Williamson, D. (2013). Vaccine delivery using nanoparticles. *Frontiers in Cellular and Infection Microbiology*, 3. https://doi:10.3389/fcimb.2013.00013, ISSN 2235-2988.

Petkar, K. C., Patil, S. M., Chavhan, S. S., Kaneko, K., Sawant, K. K., Kunda, N. K., & Saleem, I. Y. (2021). An overview of nanocarrier-based adjuvants for vaccine delivery. *Pharmaceutics*, 13(4), 455. https://doi.org/10.3390/pharmaceutics13040455.

Schmidt, S., Pedersen, G., & Christensen, D. (2018). Rational design and in vivo characterization of vaccine adjuvants. *ILAR Journal*, 59, 309–322. https://doi.org/10.1093/ilar/ily018.

Wang, N., Qian, R., Liu, T., Wu, T., & Wang, T. (2019). Nanoparticulate carriers used as vaccine adjuvant delivery systems. *Critical Reviews in Therapeutic Drug Carrier Systems*, 36(5), 449–484. https://doi.org/10.1615/CritRevTherDrugCarrierSyst.2019027047.

10 Future of Nanomedicine and Drug Delivery System

10.1 INTRODUCTION

Scientists are increasingly interested in nanomedicines for a variety of medical applications. Encompassing more effective drug delivery and targeting, as well as personalized nanomedicine, which administers a drug to a patient based on their genetic profile. Nanotherapeutics are increasingly being commercialized around the world. North America and Europe currently dominate the global nanomedicine market, owing to their superior number of patented nanotherapeutics and favorable regulatory frameworks. However, with the recent increase in the number of nanomedical research grants in Asia and the increased demand for improved disease treatments, Asia's nanotechnology-based healthcare industry is rapidly expanding. A large number of nanotherapeutics have received commercialization approval or are in clinical trials.

It is inevitable that nanomedicines outperform conventional medicines in evaluating the efficacy, bioavailability, improved transport across biological barriers and disease targeting, improved adsorption, sustained circulation and blood concentration, lower toxicity and immunogenicity, and so on. These characteristics, which are determined by their basic physicochemical properties, such as size, surface/volume ratio, softness/hardness, and surface characteristics, have improved the lives of many patients. Nonetheless, a thorough physicochemical characterization of the nanomedicine before an in vivo evaluation is one of the requirements for progress in this field. When research is carried out in accordance with proper standards and controls, valuable knowledge is accumulated for the benefit of the entire scientific establishment. While regulatory agency guidance is necessary for detecting the information required for new drug applications (NDAs), the diverse nature of various nanomedicine approaches have hampered the realization of a general guidance protocol.

Emerging nanoparticles such as block copolymer micelles, polymers, carbon nanotubes, quantum dots, and dendrimers are intended to aid in the delivery or targeting of drugs.

Carbon nanotubes are being studied not only for their potential applications in therapy, particularly cancer treatment but also for the development of new diagnostic agents and nanosensors. Carbon nanotubes can be used to deliver drugs to specific locations. Quantum dots can be used for the drug carriers or fluorescent labels for other drug carriers like liposomes. They can facilitate the creation of therapeutic strategies for cancer by combining molecular imaging for diagnostics with therapy.

DOI: 10.1201/9781003252122-10

Toxicology is a major concern for both carbon nanotubes and quantum dots, and researchers are working on ways to make these substances less hazardous before including them in medical applications.

Dendrimers are molecules with a tree-like structure that is regular and highly branched. They have a hydrophobic internal cavity that can be filled with hydrophobic molecules such as anticancer drugs and they measure between 1 and 10 nm in diameter. Dendrimers are mechanically more stable than other drug carriers, such as liposomes, but can only carry a fraction of the drug.

10.2 CHALLENGES IN NANO-BASED DRUG FORMULATIONS

- A detailed assessment of the safety of nanotherapeutics is necessary for clinical translation, but currently there is a lack of methods and standards for evaluation of the safety of nanodrugs. Methods used for traditional drugs cannot accurately evaluate the safety of nanotherapeutics. Physicochemical properties such as size, morphology, surface area, and aggregation induced at larger scales may alter biodistribution and interactions with cells and biomolecules, complicating safety issues.
- Biological challenges for nanotherapeutic development mainly involve the drug biodistribution and biological barriers. The biological fates of nanotherapeutics determine their clinical utility. Therefore, biodistribution modulation has become a focus of attention in drug development, and it aims at enhancing the accumulation of drug at the target site and reducing accumulation in healthy tissue. Biodistribution is affected by interactions with biological barriers, both external (skin, organ) and internal (cellular) barriers. Therefore, the interaction between nanotherapeutics and biological barriers during drug transport must be well characterized, as well as the impacts of transport efficiency and targeting on the safety and efficacy of the nanotherapeutics. Another biological challenge is the heterogeneity of human disease and differences between animals and humans that impact biodistribution and become apparent in clinical studies.
- Large-scale synthesis of nanotherapeutics with high repeatability is crucial for clinical translation. Many nanotherapeutics fail to enter the market because they do not meet the requirements of scale-up synthesis and reproducibility. Challenges in large-scale drug preparation are greater for nanotherapeutics due to their complexity. It is easier to control and optimize a formulation when using small batches; in contrast, in large-scale production, slight variations in the manufacturing process can result in large, critical changes in physicochemical properties such as drug composition, size, surface charge, crystallinity, and even therapeutic outcomes. Furthermore, scale-up of nanotherapeutics often requires large costs which can prevent the success of a novel nanotherapeutic. In addition to the manufacturing cost, the cost of preclinical and clinical development is also increasing. Acquiring regulatory approval is difficult for new nanotherapeutics, especially when existing products on the market have the same target indication.

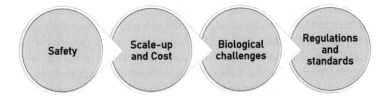

FIGURE 10.1   Common challenges in nanomedicine.

- The lack of regulation and standards for nanotherapeutics in manufacturing practices, quality control, safety, and efficacy evaluation are a barrier for the development of nanotherapeutics. There are currently no global regulatory standards specific to clinical translation of nanotherapeutics. Only initial guidance documents for nanotechnology products have been issued by regulatory authorities such as the FDA and European Medicines Agency (EMA) to provide guidance (Pasut, 2019) (Figure 10.1).

10.3   FUTURE DEMANDS FOR NANOMEDICINE RESEARCH

The incorporation of nanotechnology into conventional drugs has the potential to improve their treatment effectiveness. Many nanotherapeutics, conversely, cannot avoid triggering damage to healthy tissues because they really do not have specifically target lesions. One of the top priorities for the next generation of nanotherapeutics is to develop particular, high-efficiency drugs that hoard in lesions rather than healthy non-target tissues. Smart drug delivery systems with active targeting and stimuli responsiveness have recently been developed. These smart drug delivery systems represent a promising strategy for eliminating pathological tissues while protecting normal tissues, and they represent both a valuable opportunity and a significant challenge for the future development of nanomedicine (Zhang et al., 2020).

I. **Enhanced Passive Targeting to Pathological Tissues:** Passive targeting refers the preferential accumulation of drugs in pathological tissues such as tumors and inflamed tissues by the enhanced permeability and retention (EPR) effect, in which the leaky vasculature of tumors allows greater drug entry, or by an EPR-like effect, in which inflamed tissues release vasodilators and chemotactic factors that promote drug uptake. Therefore, strategies have been developed to improve the half-life while also enhancing the intratumoral penetration depth of nanodrugs. For example, stimuli-responsive NPs that change in size in response to changes in their environment have been developed. These NPs are large when administered and achieve longer half-lives and enhanced passive targeting to tumors via the EPR effect. After reaching the tumor microenvironment (TME), the stimuli-responsive NPs transform into small NPs, promoting penetration of the NPs into the tumor. Other strategies have also been developed to promote tumor penetration of nanotherapeutics, including penetration-enhancing ligands, modulating the TME, and other mechanisms of controlled drug release in tumors. Further investigation is needed for clinical translation of these strategies.

II. **Enhanced Active Targeting to Pathological Tissues:** Active-targeting nanotherapeutics can achieve site-specific delivery by presenting targeting ligands on their surface that recognize receptors overexpressed in pathological tissues, facilitating selective drug uptake. Although both passive and active targeting exploit the EPR effect to achieve drug accumulation in target tissues, active targeting enhances cell internalization at target sites and reduces the amount of drug exposure to healthy tissue. Most targets used currently also exist in healthy, non-cancer tissues. Furthermore, uptake of nanotherapeutics by solid tumors and the resulting therapeutic efficacy for solid tumors remain limited. Therefore, active-targeting nanotherapeutics that can deeply penetrate solid tumors should be further developed.

III. **Stimuli-Responsive Drug Delivery Systems:** Stimuli-responsive nanotherapeutics that allow triggered drug release have been developed to achieve more precise and effective cancer therapy. Stimuli-responsive anticancer nanotherapeutics have demonstrated improved therapeutic efficacy in preclinical studies, and they have demonstrated controlled drug release by both endogenous and exogenous stimuli. However, clinical translation of stimuli-responsive drug delivery systems has been slow due to their complex design, which leads to challenges in optimization, reproducibility, and quality assurance.

10.4   CONCLUSIONS

Because of the advantages of nanotherapeutics in pharmacokinetics, therapeutic efficacy, and safety, the nanopharmaceutical industry has experienced rapid growth and development over the last decade. Nanotherapeutic research is prospering, as evidenced by the rapidly increasing number of publications in nanomedicine. More importantly, many nanotherapeutics, including polymeric, liposomal, nanocrystal, protein-based, and inorganic nanodrugs, have been approved for clinical use or are being studied in clinical trials. Nanotherapeutics present enormous opportunities, but they also present greater challenges than traditional drugs. Although traditional drugs continue to dominate the market, nanotechnologies are increasingly being used to reduce side effects and improve efficacy. Nanotherapeutics, for example, will play a critical role in promoting the prevalent use of biotechnologies such as gene therapy. Nanotherapeutics are an ideal platform for the advancement of classical pharmaceuticals.

REFERENCES

Pasut, G. (2019). Grand challenges in nano-based drug delivery. *Frontiers in Medical Technology*, 1. doi:10.3389/fmedt.2019.00001.

Zhang, C., Yan, L., Wang, X., Zhu, S., Chen, C., Gu, Z., & Zhao, Y. (2020). Progress, challenges, and future of nanomedicine. *Nano Today*, 35, 101008. doi:10.1016/j.nantod.2020.101008.

Index

Verlag GmbH, Kaulbachstraße 2A, 80333 München, Germany

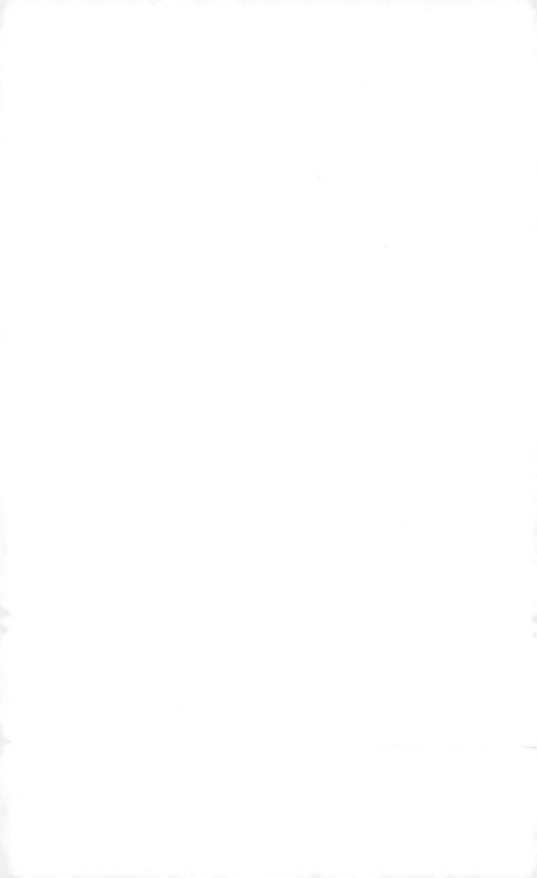